Chronotherapeutics for Affective Disorders

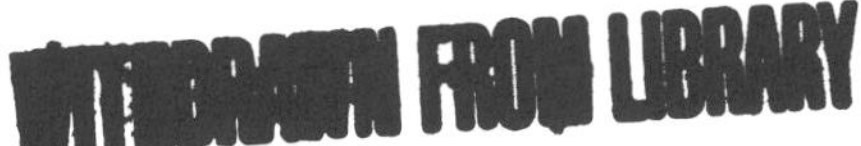

Supported by a grant from the

VELUX STIFTUNG
www.veluxstiftung.ch

Dedicated to research in the areas of daylight, medicine and biology, and the preservation of the ecological stability of nature.

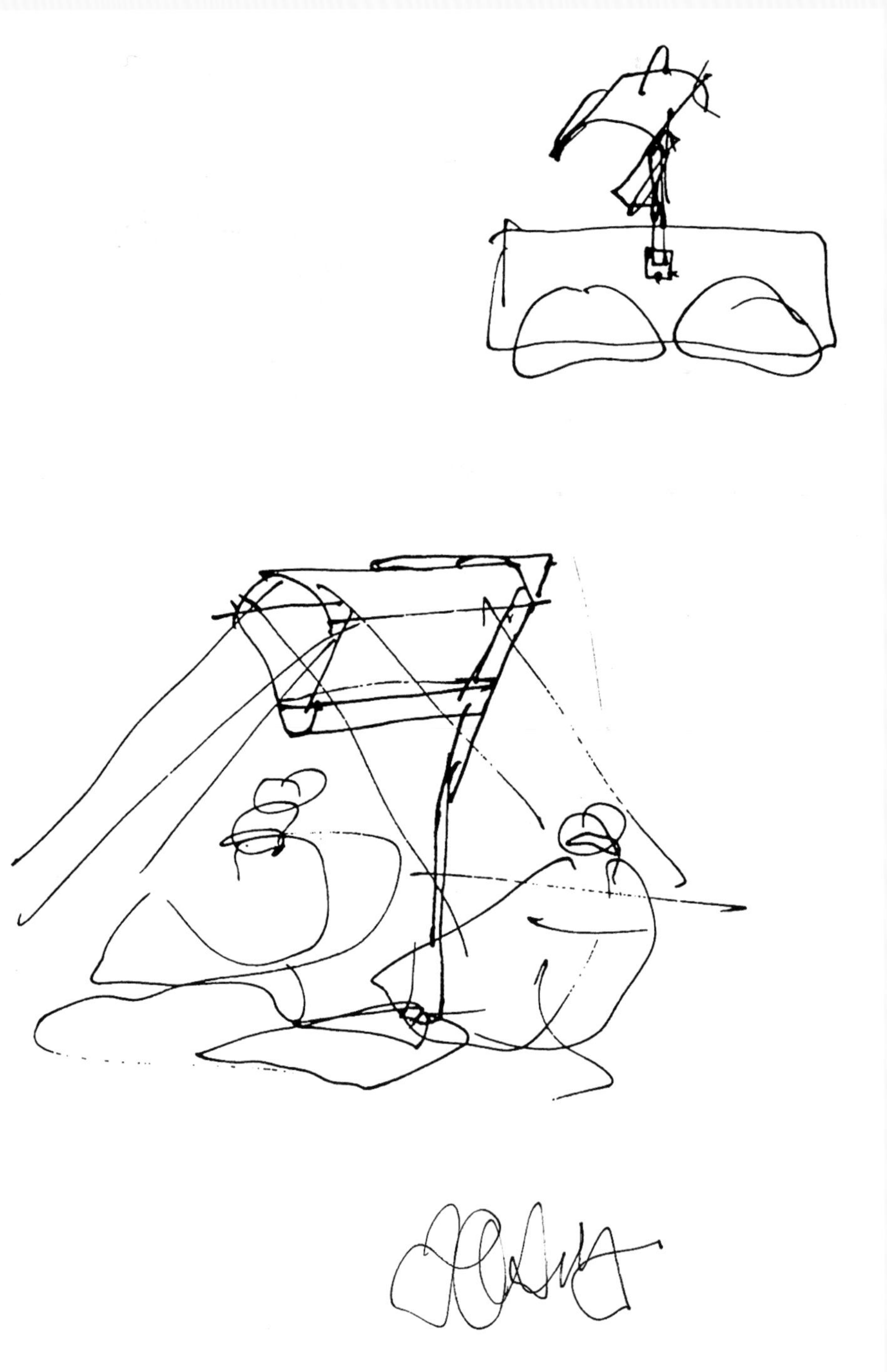

Frank Gehry (from a studio work session with Michael Terman, Santa Monica, Calif., USA, 1988).
Visions of Bedroom Dawn Simulation and Bright Light Therapy.

Anna Wirz-Justice
Francesco Benedetti
Michael Terman

Chronotherapeutics for Affective Disorders

A Clinician's Manual for Light and Wake Therapy

33 figures, 21 in color, 10 tables, 2009

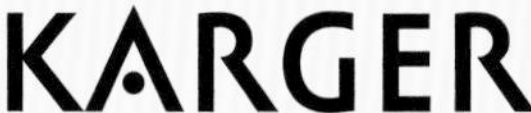

Basel · Freiburg · Paris · London · New York · Bangalore · Bangkok · Shanghai · Singapore · Tokyo · Sydney

Anna Wirz-Justice
Centre for Chronobiology
Psychiatric University Clinics
Basel, Switzerland

Francesco Benedetti
Department of Clinical Neurosciences
Scientific Institute and
University Vita-Salute San Raffaele
Milano, Italy

Michael Terman
Department of Psychiatry
Columbia University
New York, N.Y., USA

A project of the

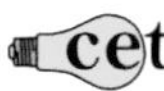

Center for Environmental Therapeutics
www.cet.org

An independent, non-profit
professional agency dedicated to education and
research on the new environmental therapies.

Library of Congress Cataloging-in-Publication Data

Wirz-Justice, Anna.
Chronotherapeutics for affective disorders : a clinician's manual for light and wake therapy / Anna Wirz-Justice, Francesco Benedetti, Michael Terman.
p. ; cm.
Includes bibliographical references and index.
ISBN 978-3-8055-9120-1 (pbk. : alk. paper)
1. Affective disorders--Alternative treatment. 2. Clinical chronobiology. 3. Circadian rhythms--Therapeutic use. 4. Sleep deprivation--Therapeutic use. 5. Light--Therapeutic use. I. Benedetti, Francesco, 1966- II. Terman, Michael. III. Title.
[DNLM: 1. Mood Disorders--therapy. 2. Chronotherapy--methods. 3. Phototherapy--methods. 4. Sleep Disorders--therapy. WM 171 W799c 2009]
RC537.W575 2009
616.85'2706--dc22
2009000805

www.karger.com
Printed in Switzerland on acid-free and non-aging paper (ISO 9706) by Reinhardt Druck, Basel
ISBN 978–3–8055–9120–1
e-ISBN 978–3–8055–9121–8

Contents

Indications

Pharmacology

Future Prospects

Foreword

Sun worship has existed since the beginning of human life on earth. Light is our source of energy, of warmth, of spiritual and emotional sustenance. Light is the major synchroniser of the biological clock. It is no surprise to see light enter psychiatry as a practical treatment. Sleep deprivation has been investigated for three decades: the instantaneous, overnight remission of severe depression remains one of the most striking phenomena in psychiatry. Sleep deprivation did not enter the therapeutic armamentarium because patients usually relapse after recovery sleep, or even a nap. Now we have learned how to sustain the effect with morning light therapy, sleep phase advances and a variety of medications. Practical experience shows that major depression can indeed remit quickly and remain remitted even in otherwise refractory cases.

Here, we combine the elements of chronotherapeutics in a new synthesis. We hope that the methods will be widely explored on inpatient units, with the prospect of higher success rates, real remissions without ominous residual symptoms, and shorter hospital stays.

We designed this manual as a source book for clinicians. Readers can choose which category to read. We begin by presenting the insights of chronobiology and sleep research that provide the scientific basis, followed by an overview of the clinical literature, which justifies the treatments (Background). We then describe the principal therapeutic procedures with practical details for both inpatients and outpatients, and for younger and older individuals (Methods). Beyond the core depressive disorders, we consider a broader range of current and potential applications (Indications), introduce melatonin and drugs that affect rhythms (Pharmacology), ending with a discussion of social issues that impinge on rhythmic structure and everyday well-being (Future Prospects).

Outpatients with affective disorders can learn to use light therapy – and even wake therapy – at home, but they must have directive coaching by the clinician. The current mode – 'Go buy/try a light box, see if it works. (Period.)' – is a formula for disappointment, and discredits the solid clinical research of more than 20 years. Clinicians need to learn the timing principles of the circadian clock's response to light, and carefully dose the treatment as they would a medication.

Not to give up medication, though: the combination of light therapy with antidepressants can provide a potent enhancement over either one alone. The lucky minority – as we have seen in seasonal depression – will be able to taper drugs to discontinuation and remain euthymic under maintenance light monotherapy.

A new therapeutic paradigm often seeks a new generation of clinicians, and we especially encourage psychiatric residents to get these principles under their belt – to help the field identify limitations and refinements, and to view each case as an important learning experience for all of us. As we emphasize in the Manual, there are significant loose ends that can and should be resolved before we contemplate a second, revised edition. Feedback from the field is now our priority.

In 1988, a cloistered group of about 100 circadian rhythm aficionados and psychiatrists founded the Society for Light Treatment and Biological Rhythms (www.sltbr.org), with an annual summer scientific meeting including clinical trial reports, animal model studies, basic research in relevant photobiology, CME courses, contentious debates, and consensus development. If this Manual stimulates you, you should join SLTBR, follow its online news, and come to the annual meeting to share your experiences and help the field grow.

Also, we encourage readers to join a 'members-only' web forum on chronotherapeutics by accessing http://www.chronotherapeutics.org and registering with the password 'colleagues'.

Anna Wirz-Justice, Basel
Francesco Benedetti, Milano
Michael Terman, New York

Acknowledgements

This book is dedicated to our teachers and colleagues, past and present, whose scientific acumen led to a fusion of biological and clinical insight that sparked the development of chronotherapeutics in psychiatry:

Josephine Arendt
Jürgen Aschoff
Domien Beersma
Mathias Berger
Alexander Borbély
William Bunney, Jr.
Serge Daan
Charmane Eastman
Russell Foster
Christian Gillin
Frederick Goodwin
Günter Hole
Siegfried Kasper
Donald Klein
Daniel Kripke
Alfred Lewy
Kazuo Mishima
Masako Okawa
Dan Oren
Herbert Pardes
Barbara Parry
Burkard Pflug
Colin Pittendrigh
Robert Post
Charlotte Remé
Till Roenneberg
Norman Rosenthal
Robert Spitzer
Jonathan Stewart
Kiyohisa Takahashi
Rütger van den Hoofdakker
Eus van Someren
Thomas Wehr
Rütger Wever
Peter Whybrow
Janet Williams
Richard Wurtman
Martin Zatz
Irving Zucker

With appreciation for our coworkers and their major contributions to the underlying studies:

Janis Anderson
Barbara Barbini
Christian Cajochen
Cristina Colombo
Konstantin Danilenko
Wallace Duncan
Stephen Fairhurst
Namni Goel
Marijke Gordijn
Hans-Joachim Haug
Kurt Kräuchi
Raymond Lam
Klaus Martiny
Patrick McGrath
Brian Rafferty
Donald Ross
Dorothy Sit
Enrico Smeraldi
Milica Stefanovik
Jonathan Stewart
Jiuan Su Terman
Thomas White
Katherine Wisner
Joseph Wu

Special thanks to Jiuan Su Terman for her critical review of the manuscript.

We are grateful to our institutions for their steadfast support of risky innovation: Psychiatric University Clinics Basel, Switzerland; Scientific Institute and University Vita-Salute San Raffaele, Milano, Italy; and Columbia University Department of Psychiatry, New York, N.Y., USA.

Our research was supported by the National Institute of Mental Health (USA), the Swiss National Science Foundation, the Velux Stiftung, EU FP6 integrated project 'EUCLOCK', and by our institutions.

Royalties for this manual are directed to CET's initiatives in environmental therapeutics.

List of Abbreviations

5HT	Serotonin
AD	Alzheimer's dementia
ADHD	Attention deficit/hyperactivity disorder
ARMD	Age-related macular degeneration
ASPD	Advanced sleep phase disorder
BP	Bipolar disorder
CET	Center for Environmental Therapeutics
CT	Circadian time (vs. solar time)
DDS	Dawn-dusk simulation/simulator
DLMO	Dim light melatonin onset
DSM-IV	Diagnostic and Statistical Manual of Mental Disorders, ed 4
DSPD	Delayed sleep phase disorder
ECT	Electroconvulsive therapy
GABA	Gamma-aminobutyric acid
HAMD	Hamilton Depression Rating Scale
IGL	Intergeniculate leaflet
IPSRT	Interpersonal social rhythm therapy
ISAD	International Society for Affective Disorders
lx	Lux (illuminance)
MAOA	Monoamine oxidase-A
MEQ	Morningness-Eveningness (chronotype) Questionnaire
MT1	Melatonin 1 receptor
MT2	Melatonin 2 receptor
NA	Noradrenaline
NLP	No conscious light perception (sensory blindness)
PMDD	Premenstrual dysphoric disorder
PMS	Premenstrual syndrome
PVN	Paraventricular nucleus
PWT	Partial wake therapy (second half of the night)
RHT	Retinohypothalamic tract
SAD	Seasonal affective disorder
SCN	Suprachiasmatic nuclei of the hypothalamus
SD	Sleep deprivation
SIGH-ADS	Structured Interview for the Hamilton Depression Scale with Atypical Depression Supplement
SSRI	Selective serotonin reuptake inhibitor
TCA	Tricyclic antidepressant
UV	Ultraviolet radiation
UVA	UV radiation band closest to the visible (violet/blue) spectrum
WT	Wake therapy (whole night plus day before and after)

1

Introduction

This Manual is written for psychiatrists, psychologists, primary care physicians, nurses, and all persons involved in treating patients with major depression (unipolar and bipolar) in a clinical or ambulatory setting. The aim is first, to present the theory behind these non-pharmaceutical chronobiological treatments; second, to document the evidence that they are efficacious in controlled trials, and third, to provide a handbook for step-by-step implementation of these therapies in everyday practice. The theoretical chapters can be skipped, and the interventions still be effectively applied. Selected references focus on new reviews and clinically relevant studies that will lead the reader to the original research.

1.1 Unmet Needs in the Treatment of Depression

Much progress has been made in dissecting the *Anatomy of Melancholy* since Robert Burton wrote his extensive treatise in 1621 (fig. 1). Those involved in treating patients with depression know that we have many evidence-based treatments, from psychotherapy to psychopharmacology. Important developments in the treatment of major depression over the last decades include cognitive behavioural therapy, SSRIs, and mixed NA/5HT reuptake inhibitors, both with a better side-effect profile than the classic tricyclics. Yet we have not attained our goal, the right treatment for every patient and the minimisation of residual symptoms. None of these treatments has broken the time barrier with fast onset of action, which remains the crux for clinicians who need to carefully monitor patients in the critical period until antidepressants begin to work. The slow action of antidepressants is particularly worrisome for severely depressed or suicidal patients. Furthermore, not all patients respond to all drugs, and it usually takes an odyssey through various medications and their combinations to find the right mix. And, although responding, many patients show residual symptoms – which increases the risk of relapse.

There is an intensive search for new psychopharmacologic agents. Antidepressants based on classic neurotransmitter systems are still a prime focus, but there are many novel drug targets other than monoamines. Strategies that promote adjuvant therapy are on the increase, whether a combination with other medications (e.g. pindolol, thyroid hormone) or psychological interventions (e.g. cognitive behavioural therapy).

We already have the means to speed up response without waiting for that miracle drug – or using the most powerful and rapid, yet unwieldy tool, electroconvulsive therapy (ECT). Chronobiological treatments are well tested and efficacious. They can be combined with any medication conventionally used for major depression. Light therapy has undergone widespread controlled, randomised clinical trials, particularly – but not only – in seasonal affective disorder (SAD). Light therapy is accepted worldwide as the treatment of choice for SAD; recent research focus has moved to non-seasonal depression, where studies are now showing that adjuvant light induces faster and greater antidepressant response.

Sleep deprivation has been widely studied for more than three decades. Were sleep deprivation an easily-administered pill, it would be the treatment of choice for major depression, with an amazing onset of action within hours in approxi-

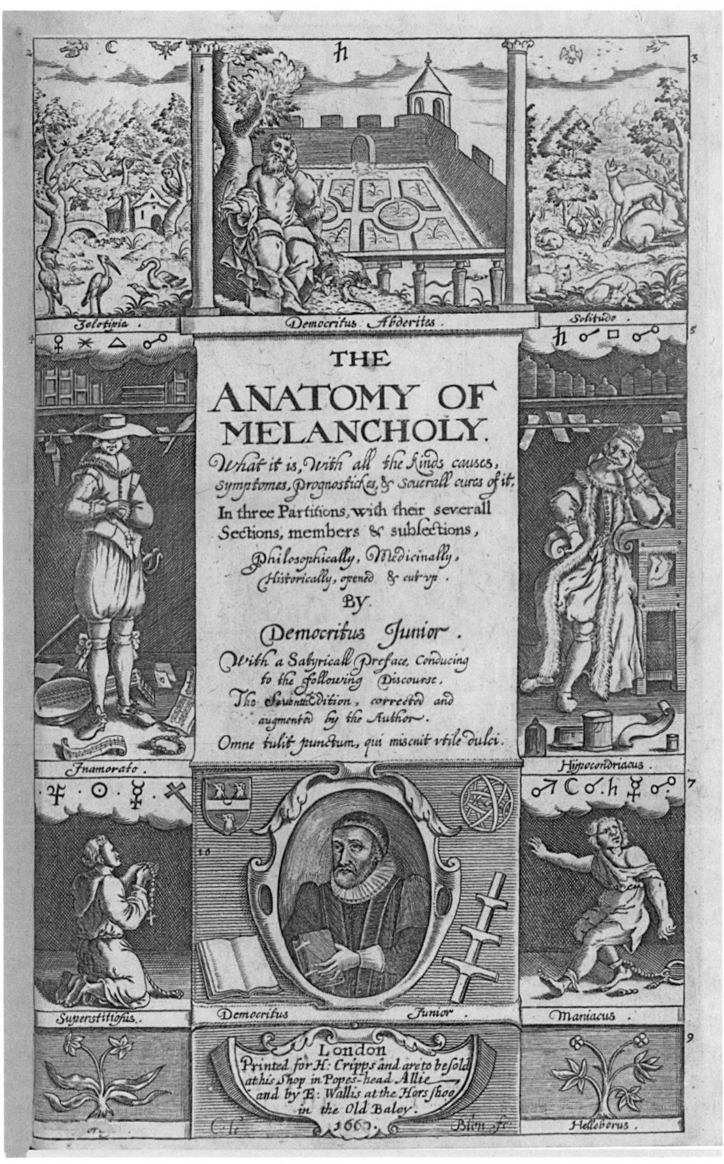

Fig. 1. Frontispiece of Robert Burton's *The Anatomy of Melancholy*, ed. 7, 1660.

mately 60% of patients. The data documenting its efficacy – gathered mostly in Europe – are unambiguous, convincing and replicable. There are several reasons why this therapy has not been incorporated into everyday psychiatric practice. One is psychological: the patient who suffers insomnia is asked to remain without sleep – is this a joke, a torture, or ignorance of the miseries of the sleep disturbances intrinsic to depression? If one changed the name, would the attitude and acceptance change? Would we enthusiastically treat patients with 'wake therapy' even though we shy from attempting 'sleep deprivation'?

Combining these methods with medication has hardly been tried. There has been no consensus development and no lobby for widespread education and application. It may be because companies cannot patent these treatments – there is no profit motive. These non-pharmaceutical, biologically based therapies are not only powerful adjuvants, but also antidepressants in their own right. We have a responsibility to offer them to our patients. There are practically no side effects, they are cost-effective, and we expect that they will shorten the length of hospitalisation.

The International Society for Affective Disorders (ISAD) convened a Committee on Chronotherapeutics to review chronobiologic treatments for depression (https://www.isad.org.uk/committees/chrono_therapy.asp). The report was published as an editorial in *Psychological Medicine* [1]. The recommendations are summarised in table 1, the list of chronotherapeutic modalities in table 2.

This Manual provides theoretical and practical guidelines for implementing wake therapy and light treatment in clinical practice. It fulfils an objective of our non-profit organisation (Center for Environmental Therapeutics, www.cet.org) to provide research-based, reliable information about these non-pharmacologic treatments. While our focus is on hospitalised patients, light therapy is easily applied to outpatients, and wake therapy can be offered in ambulatory centres (section 7).

Table 1. Recommendations of the Committee on Chronotherapeutics of the International Society for Affective Disorders (ISAD) [1]

1	Sleep deprivation (wake therapy) is the most rapid antidepressant available today: approximately 60% of patients, independent of diagnostic subtype, respond with marked improvement within hours. Treatment can be a single or repeated sleep deprivation, total (all night) or partial (second half of the night). Relapse can be prevented by daily light therapy, concomitant administration of SSRIs, lithium (for bipolar patients), or a short phase advance of sleep over 3 days following a single night of wake therapy. Combinations of these interventions show great promise.
2	Light therapy is effective for major depression – not only for the seasonal subtype. As an adjuvant to conventional antidepressants in unipolar patients, or lithium in bipolar patients, morning light hastens and potentiates the antidepressant response. Light therapy shows benefit even for patients with chronic depression of 2 years or more, outperforming their weak response to drugs. This method provides a viable alternative for patients who refuse, resist or cannot tolerate medication, or for whom drugs may be contraindicated, as in antepartum depression.
3	Given the urgent need for new strategies to treat patients with residual depressive symptoms, clinical trials of wake therapy and/or adjuvant light therapy, coupled with follow-up studies of long-term recurrence, are a high priority.

Table 2. Circadian and wake therapies for major depression

	Therapeutic response	
	latency	duration
Total sleep deprivation = wake therapy (WT)	hours	~1 day
Partial sleep deprivation 2nd half of the night (PWT)	hours	~1 day
Repeated WT or PWT	hours	days/weeks
Repeated WT or PWT with antidepressants	hours	weeks/months
Phase advance of the sleep-wake cycle	~3 days	1–2 weeks
WT followed by sleep phase advance	hours	1–3 weeks
Single/repeated WT or PWT + light therapy	hours	weeks
Single/repeated WT or PWT + phase advance + light therapy	hours	weeks
Single/repeated WT or PWT + lithium, pindolol, or SSRIs	hours	months
Light therapy (winter seasonal depression)	days	weeks/months
Light therapy (nonseasonal depression)	weeks	weeks/months
Light therapy + SSRIs (nonseasonal depression)	1–2 weeks	weeks/months
Dark or rest therapy for mania or rapid cycling	days	throughout maintenance of treatment

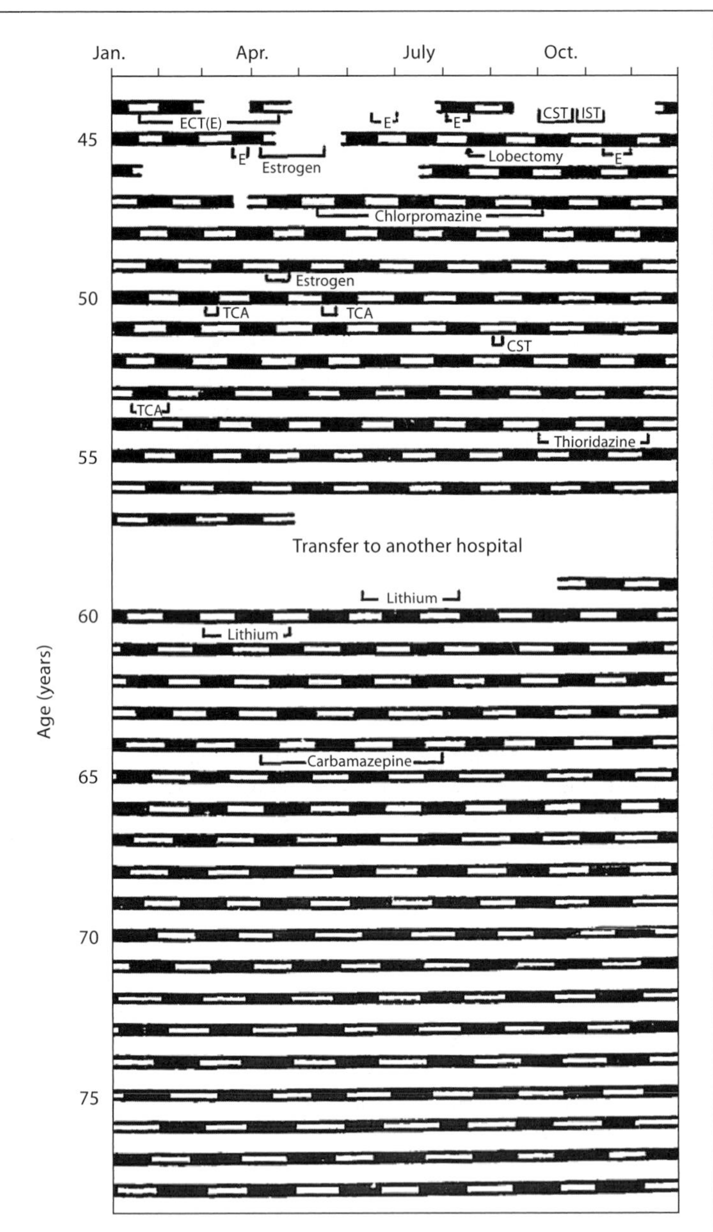

Fig. 2. Clinical record (35 years) of a rapid-cycling bipolar woman with 2- to 4-day cycles of depression (black bars) and mania (white bars). No drug treatment affected the periodicity. CST = Continuous sleep therapy; IST = insulin shock therapy; TCA = tricyclic antidepressant. From Mizukawa et al. [3], with permission.

1.2 Role of Biological Rhythms in Psychiatry

One of the most striking clinical phenomena in affective disorders is its periodicity – ranging from seasonal, as in winter depression, to rapid cycling [3] (fig. 2), which can be as short as 48 h. Other periodic phenomena are found at the symptom level: diurnal variation of mood, early morning awakening and sleep disturbances. A great deal of research has documented abnormal circadian rhythms in biochemistry, neuroendo-

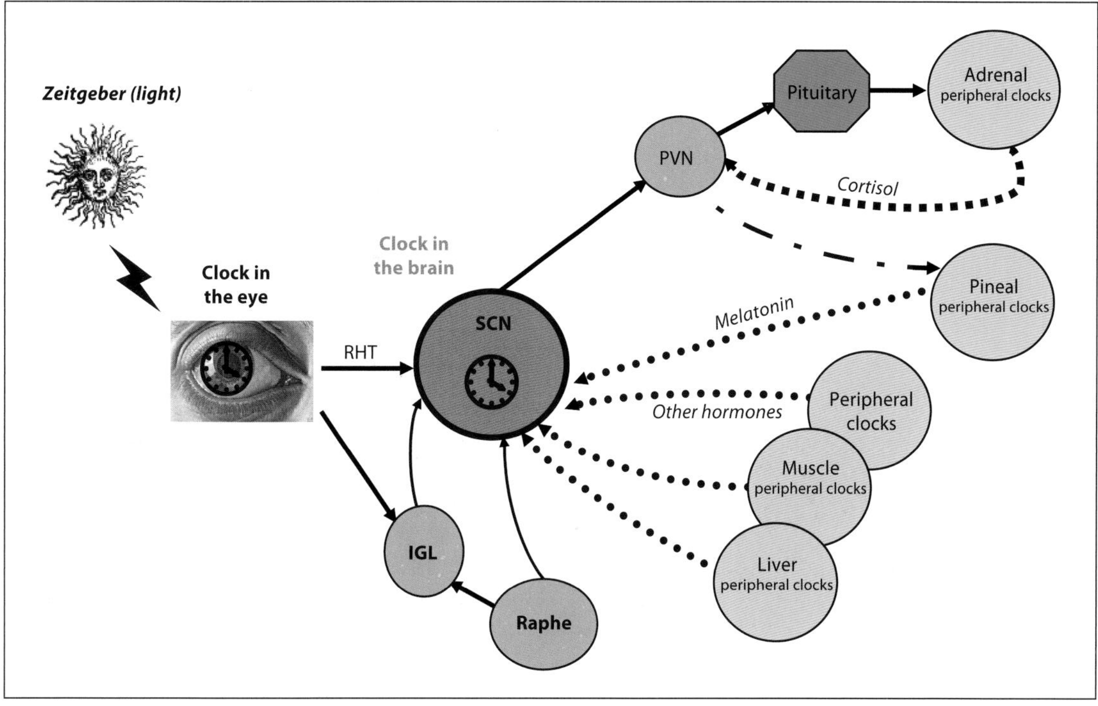

Fig. 3. Schematic representation of the circadian timing system. Light is the primary zeitgeber ('time-giver' or synchronising agent) for the biological clock in the SCN, via specialised circadian photoreceptors in the retina. A multisynaptic pathway to the pineal gland drives the nocturnal synthesis of melatonin and enables its suppression by light. Melatonin feeds back on receptors in the SCN. The SCN also synchronises the timing of peripheral clocks in other organs and cells, some of which have their own zeitgebers (e.g. food for the liver clock). There are multiple connections from (and to) the SCN with areas of the brain involved in sleep regulation.

crine function, physiology and behaviour in depressed patients [2]. The findings point towards increased variability in day-to-day rhythms, low circadian amplitude, and abnormal circadian timing – either too early or too late. Bipolar disorder is most clearly linked to changes in circadian timing with clinical state.

1.3 Principles of Circadian Timing

The circadian system [4] is schematically described in figure 3. A master pacemaker or biological clock in the hypothalamic suprachiasmatic nuclei (SCN) drives all circadian rhythms in the brain and body. The endogenous clock ticks at a period different from, usually slightly longer, than 24.0 h. The SCN is synchronised to the solar cycle primarily by retinal light input. This retinal signal is transmitted by a specialised ('non-visual') retino-hypothalamic tract (RHT) to the SCN. A subset of retinal ganglion cells contains the photopigment melanopsin, which responds to light energy independently of the classic photoreceptors, rods and cones [5]. While melanopsin is selectively receptive to short wavelength blue light, the cones modulate the ganglion cell response. There is strong evidence for a circadian clock in the mammalian eye as

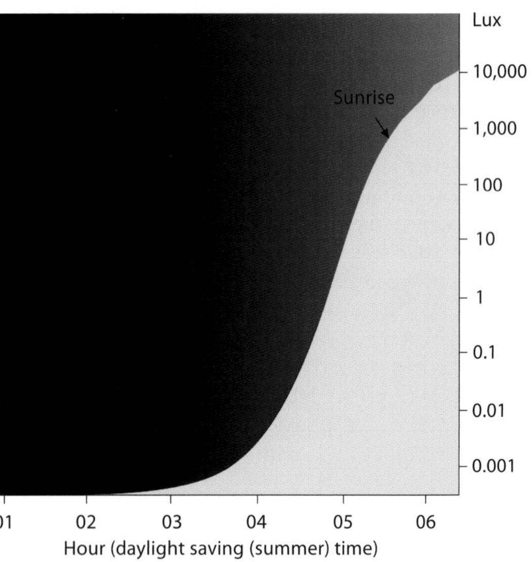

Fig. 4. Natural progression of dawn on May 5 (a typical date of spontaneous remission of winter depression). Screen shot from MacLite software used to drive dawn simulation in the bedroom. For therapeutic use, the entire curve is attenuated from 800 lx at sunrise to 300 lx or lower, depending on dose adjustment. Time of sunrise is initially adjusted to habitual wake-up time (end of subjective night) and gradually moved earlier if additional circadian rhythm phase advances are indicated (from Terman and Fairhurst, Columbia University).

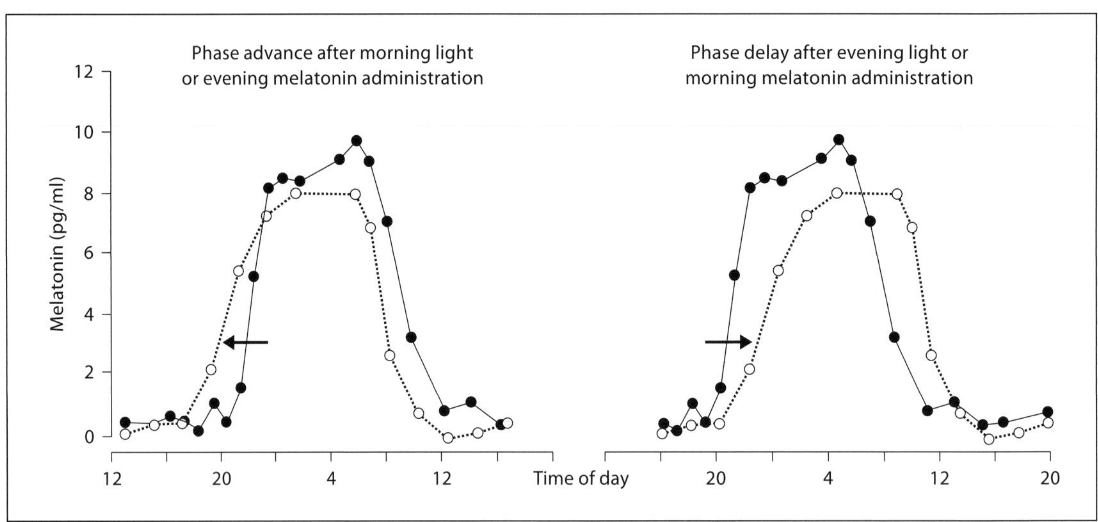

Fig. 5. Example (schematic) of a melatonin rhythm measured in saliva at baseline (full line) and after phase shifts to timed zeitgebers (light or melatonin; dotted line).

well, which rhythmically gates light input to the SCN [6, 7].

Only in the last decades has it been recognised that light is the major zeitgeber (time-giver or synchronising agent) for human circadian rhythms, being much more powerful than social zeitgebers, such as the alarm clock [8]. Environmental light spans nine orders of magnitude, from starlight to the sun overhead at midday (fig. 4). Normal room light falls into the range of civil twilight, between 100 and 300 lx. By contrast, earliest daylight with the sun rising over the

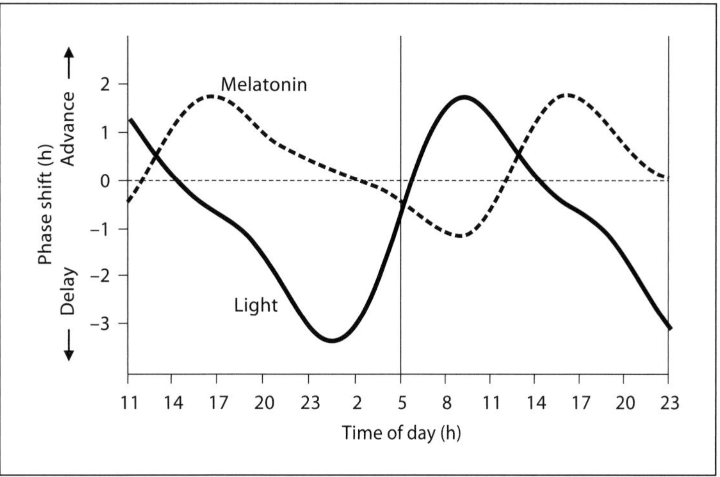

Fig. 6. Schematic representation of shifts (in hours) in the circadian system according to time of day (or circadian phase) of administration. Light (full line) given in the early morning (after the core body temperature minimum at approximately 5 a.m.) shifts the clock earlier (phase advance), in the evening (before the core body temperature minimum) to later (phase delay). Melatonin (broken line) has nearly opposite effects: morning melatonin induces a phase delay, and evening melatonin a phase advance. Redrawn from [14, 15], with permission.

horizon provides about 800 lx, and noontime light can reach 100,000 lx. Bright light therapy administers full daylight levels up to 10,000 lx, far above normal home or workplace lighting. The circadian system has evolved to respond to the natural dawn signal preceding sunrise.

Nocturnal production of the pineal hormone melatonin is driven by the SCN; melatonin also feeds back on melatonin receptors in the SCN and thus, like light, can act as a zeitgeber to phase shift and synchronise circadian rhythms [9]. As befits a 'darkness hormone', melatonin acts in a manner opposite to light. Light suppresses melatonin and thus modulates its nocturnal secretion [10]. In most mammals, melatonin acts as a seasonal signal through change in duration – long secretion in the long nights of winter, short in the short nights of summer. Moreover, when melatonin is administered before SCN-triggered pineal melatonin onset in the evening, it elicits phase advances of the circadian clock in the same manner as early morning light exposure. Conversely, when melatonin is administered in the morning, it elicits phase delays, as does evening light exposure (fig. 5).

A serotonergic pathway from the raphe nucleus provides non-photic input to the SCN [11]. Non-photic zeitgebers such as exercise, sleep or darkness are probably much weaker zeitgebers than light on SCN function [11]. Social zeitgebers (such as school or work schedules) may act directly or indirectly on the SCN, since they determine the timing of meals, sleep, physical exercise and outdoor light exposure. The circadian pacemaker has inputs to and from sleep regulatory centres [12] (section 1.4.). In addition to the primary biological clock in the SCN, we now know that circadian oscillators are found in every organ and every cell – the so-called peripheral clocks [4].

Since light and exogenously administered melatonin are major zeitgebers for the SCN, it is important to understand how they need to be administered to obtain the required result. The principle of how zeitgebers work is *timing*: the same amount of light or melatonin can shift the biological clock to earlier or later, depending on when it given. These effects are summarised in a 'phase response curve' that illustrates how much of a phase shift (advance, delay, or no effect) can be induced at different times of day (or circadian phase) (fig. 6). To shift the clock earlier, morning light and/or evening melatonin are effective [10, 13–15]; to shift to later, evening light and/or

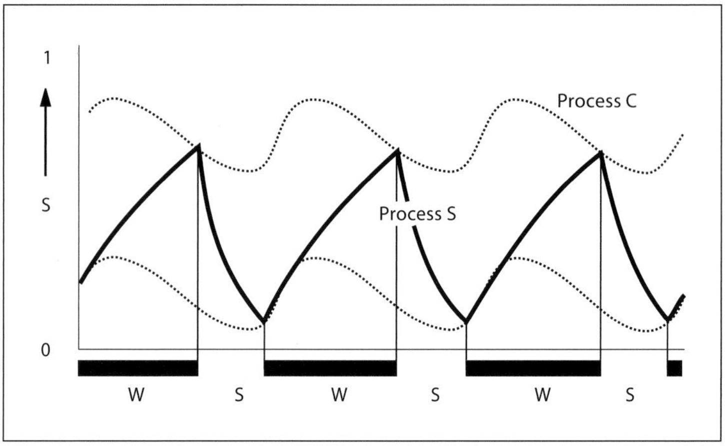

Fig. 7. Two-process model of sleep regulation. The homeostatic process S rises during wake and declines during sleep. The circadian process C (here described by two thresholds for going to and waking from sleep) determines the timing and architecture of sleep. S = Sleep; W = wake. From Daan et al. [16], with permission.

morning melatonin [10, 13–15]. Thus, timing is crucial for the optimal response. Moreover, it is important to note that a given clock time of administration is not necessarily the same 'internal clock time' for every person (particularly if circadian rhythms are disturbed, as we discuss in sections 2.2. and 4.2.).

1.4 Principles of Sleep Regulation

The timing and physiological structure of sleep are consequences of interactions between the circadian pacemaker (process C) and a homeostatic process of sleep pressure that increases with the duration of wakefulness and dissipates during sleep (process S) [16] (fig. 7). In healthy subjects, process S builds up during waking until it intersects with the phase of process C appropriate for sleep onset. Thereafter, the exponential decline, associated with slow wave sleep, intersects with the phase of process C appropriate for waking up.

It follows from this model that abnormalities in either process S or C can predispose an individual to depression [17]. For example, the normal daytime accumulation in sleep pressure may be deficient, but with sleep deprivation it will continue to accumulate over the next day. The antidepressant effect of one night without sleep (wake therapy) can be seen in terms of normalisation of process S to the usual level that precedes sleep (fig. 8). Similarly, process C can vary abnormally in phase position, oscillation amplitude, or both. These variations will determine when process S intersects the threshold for sleep onset and wake-up time (producing sleep disturbances in depressive patients, such as sleep onset insomnia with early morning awakening, or hypersomnia). Thus, the chronotherapeutic focus is on strategies that normalise process C. Appropriately timed light therapy can phase shift the circadian clock, increase its amplitude, or both (fig. 8).

1.5 Mood Level Varies with Time of Day and Duration of Wakefulness

The two-process model has been able to explain much of the physiology of sleep and wakefulness, as well as aberrant sleep-wake cycle behaviour. Beyond sleepiness per se, it is surprising to see that interactions of process C and process S regulate daily cycles of mood (clinically seen as diurnal variation) [18]. Mood follows the circadian rhythm of core body temperature rather

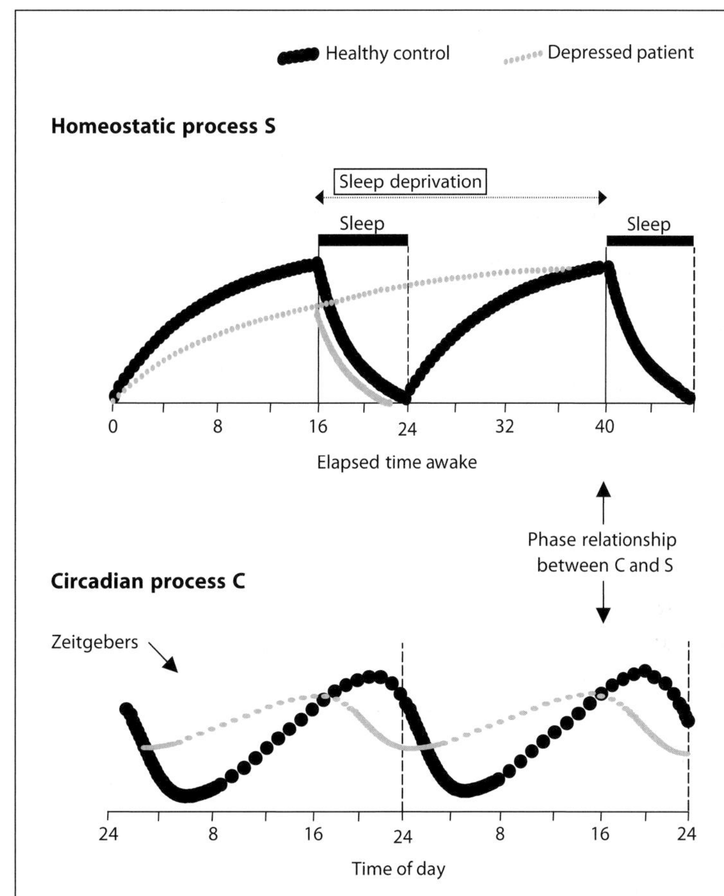

Fig. 8. The two-process model of sleep regulation as applied to depressed patients. In depression, a putative reduced or deficient level of process S is temporarily normalised by total sleep deprivation. Process C might also be modified in depression – with a lower amplitude or an earlier or later phase. The phase relationships between C and S determine the structure and stability of the sleep-wake cycle. Zeitgebers, such as light, can act both to increase amplitude and shift and stabilise phase. Redrawn from Wirz-Justice [17], with permission.

clearly. Figure 9 represents the two processes in healthy subjects, as educed components derived from a laboratory protocol [18]. Process C begins with lowest mood in the early morning, improving throughout the day with best mood in the evening, followed by a decline during the night. Process S-related mood is at its best when sleep pressure is low after awakening, and thereafter declines the longer we are awake. Normal, stable mood regulation during the day requires good temporal alignment between the sleep-wake cycle and the circadian system, so that there are no low points. By superposing and shifting these two curves around one can see how mood can drop suddenly if the two processes are not in synchrony. The consequences of misalignment are magnified for patients with depression, resulting in the clinical phenomenon of daily mood swings.

1.6 Sleep Deprivation

Oddly enough, when depressed patients stay awake for 36 h, mood does not continue to follow a linear decline as would be extrapolated from figure 9 (right). In healthy subjects, this decline occurs throughout the night, until the next day when the positive surge of the circadian system balances it.

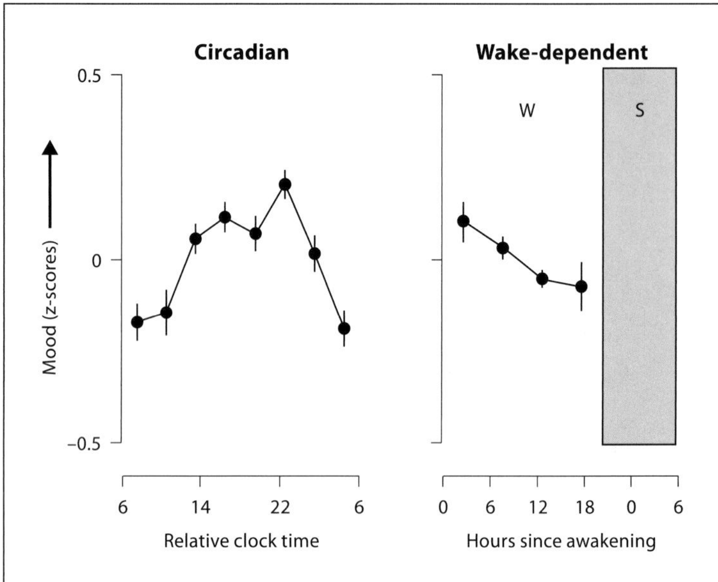

Fig. 9. The subjective rating of mood across 24 h in healthy subjects arises from an interaction between a circadian rhythm (left) and prior time spent awake (right) – here separated into the two components by means of a 'forced desynchrony' protocol. Redrawn from Boivin et al. [18], with permission.

In depression, something specific (and different from normal) is triggered by a night's sleep deprivation that leads to a profound switch in clinical state. Improvement usually begins in the second half of the night or the next day.

Many studies have documented antidepressant effects of a variety of manipulations of the sleep-wake cycle, whether of duration (total or partial sleep deprivation) or timing (partial sleep deprivation, sleep phase advance) [19–21]. The sleep manipulations are summarised in figure 10, which shows clearly that wakefulness in the latter part of the night is the key to an antidepressant response. And it is not light during the night that is inducing the antidepressant response, since patients still improve in darkness (though they find it more difficult to remain awake) [22].

1.7 How It All Began: Light Therapy for Seasonal Affective Disorder

2005 was a signal year for the field, with consensus achieved by an American Psychiatric Association work group that light can serve as a first-line treatment intervention for both seasonal and non-seasonal depression [23]. In other words, expert clinicians have judged the evidence for light therapy as a viable alternative or adjunct to antidepressant drugs [24, 25].

But how did it all begin? The diagnosis of SAD and the analogy with hamster hibernation cycles led to the development of light therapy in the early 1980s [26]. (We must note that the pharmaceutical industry has recently tried to rechristen SAD as seasonal major depressive disorder (sMDD), a misnomer which arbitrarily excises seasonal bipolar depression from the category.) The idea was simple: lengthening the daily photoperiod (in effect, mimicking summer day length) would lead to remission of winter depressive symptoms. Since that time, many centres

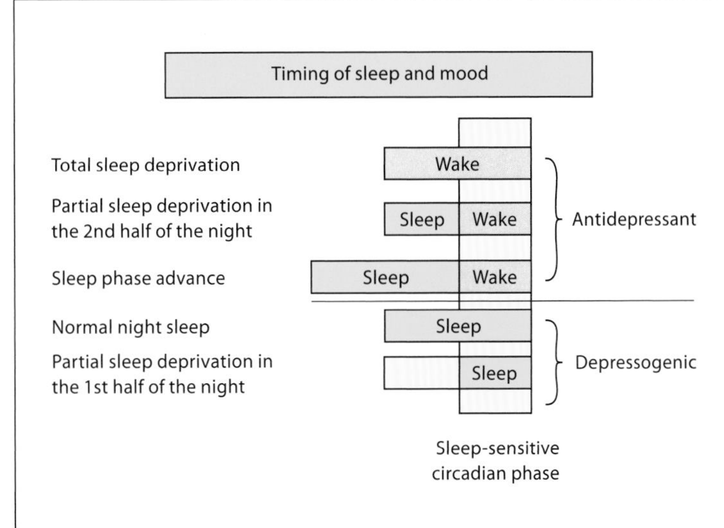

Fig. 10. Schematic representation of different manipulations of sleep timing and duration on the response of depressed patients (based on 30 years of clinical trials). A sleep-sensitive circadian phase in the second half of the night appears to be crucial in that being awake at this time can trigger improvement.

around the world have conducted studies using bright light in various protocols and applications [27, 28]. These studies have refined the clinical issues involved in use of bright light therapy, showing, for example, that it is not necessary to mimic the length of a spring or summer day for a remission of depressive symptoms, but merely to deliver the light pulse (which can be as short as 30 min) to signal a springtime sunrise to the brain. More than twenty years of clinical and neurobiological research support the diagnosis of SAD (Bipolar or Major Depressive Disorder, Recurrent, with Seasonal Pattern, by DSM-IV criteria) (table 3).

The response to light in SAD is often remarkable and consistent, as exemplified by a patient whose depression ratings were followed weekly for 4 years (fig. 11).

Table 3. Features of winter seasonal affective disorder*

- Two or more consecutive episodes of major depression in autumn or winter
- Spontaneous remission in spring or summer
- Atypical neurovegetative symptoms
  - Daytime sleepiness
  - Increased sleep need/hypersomnia
  - Increased appetite
  - Carbohydrate craving
  - Weight gain

* DSM-IV criteria do not specify atypical symptoms.

1.8 Light Therapy – Beyond SAD

Daniel Kripke was the pioneer who proposed and tested light therapy for non-seasonal depression [30, 31], but it is only now, more than 20 years later, that there are adequately controlled longer-term studies to support his predictions.

A new generation of clinical trials has begun to establish the therapeutic efficacy of light for a variety of psychiatric disorders [27, 32]. Recent double-blind, placebo-controlled studies show that light therapy combined with an SSRI leads to more rapid (within a week) and more profound (by approximately 30%) improvement in patients with non-seasonal major depression [33, 34]. The need for efficacious treatment of depression dur-

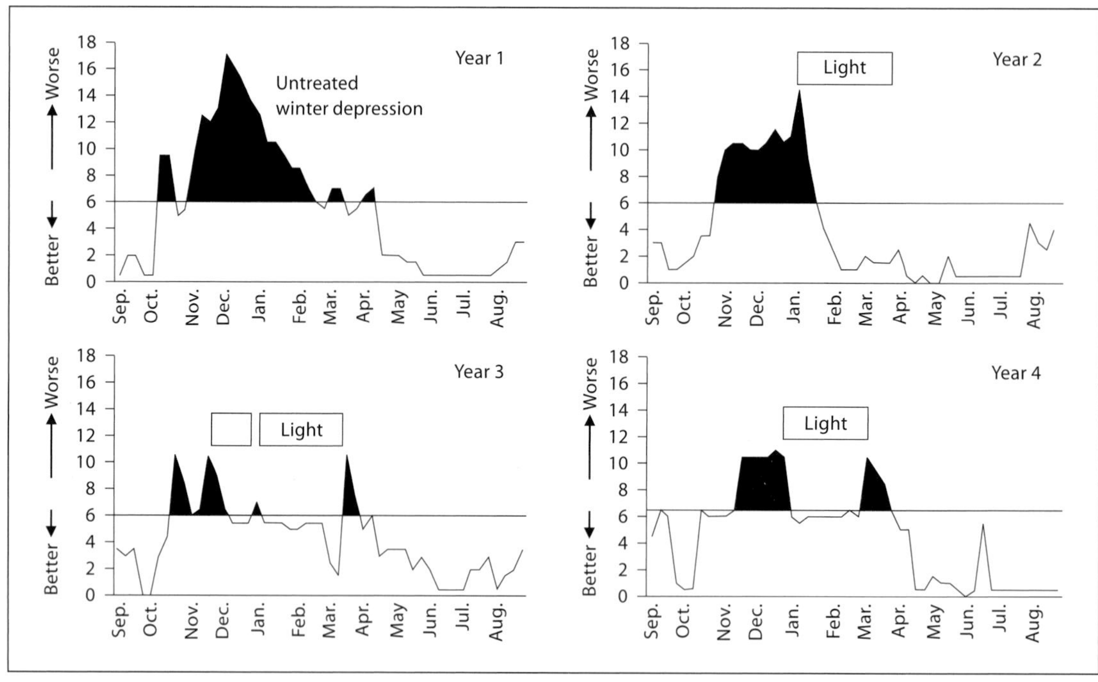

Fig. 11. Weekly depression self-ratings in a female SAD patient over 4 years (6 = threshold for depressive mood). Her winter depression episode began regularly in October. The first year illustrates the untreated natural course of the illness, with maximum depression ratings in December and January, declining to normal values in April. Light therapy begun in January of the second year induced a lasting euthymia. In year 3, light therapy began earlier, thus cutting off most of the depressive episode. Note that stopping light treatment in March resulted in a return of minor symptoms until the spontaneous remission in April. This is even more clearly seen in year 4, underlining the strongly seasonal nature of the illness. From Wirz-Justice and Staedt [29], with permission.

Table 4. Promising indications for light therapy

- SAD
- Sub-syndromal SAD
- Non-seasonal recurrent depression
- Bipolar depression
- Chronic depression
- Premenstrual dysphoric disorder
- Antepartum depression
- Attention deficit/hyperactivity disorder
- Chronic fatigue syndrome
- Schizophrenia
- Borderline personality disorder
- Parkinson's disease
- Alzheimer's disease
- Circadian rhythm sleep disorders (advanced and delayed sleep phase disorder, irregular sleep-wake cycles)

ing pregnancy without side effects for the foetus has led to trials of monotherapy with light [35]. Bulimic patients also respond to light with improvement of both depressive and bulimic symptoms [36, 37]. Light is useful in improving sleep, mood and cognition in dementia [38–40]. Most impressively, treatment of chronic depression (greater than 2 years' duration) with light has yielded impressive results in this often treatment-resistant group [41].

Thus, light is emerging as a broad-spectrum antidepressant 'drug', with an effect size equal to or better than medication, and the ability to shorten the latency to response. Even though evidence continues to accumulate in ongoing clinical trials, there is sufficient strong support for the

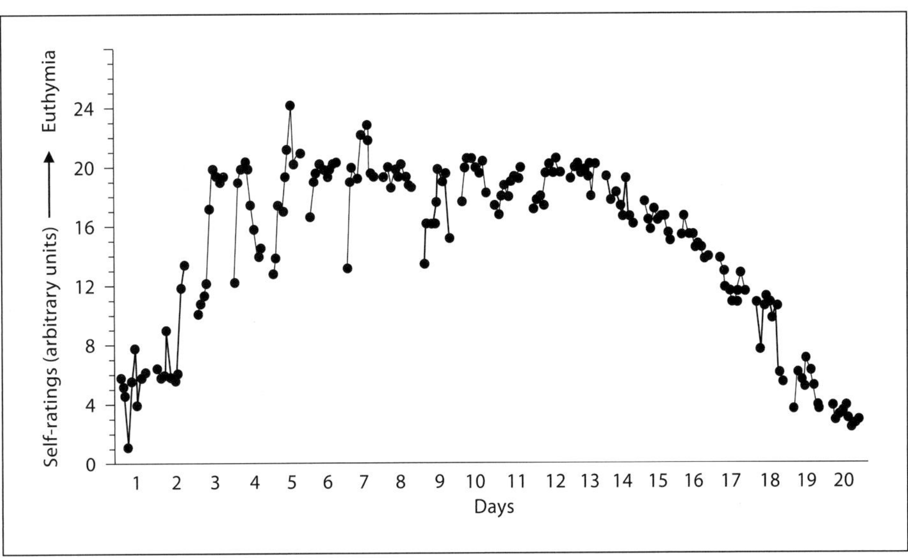

Fig. 12. Depression self-ratings every 2 h during wakefulness in a female bipolar patient whose sleep was phase advanced by 6 h to begin at 5 p.m. Over 3 weeks, overall mood rose, remained stable for a certain period, and then declined. The diurnal variation of mood showed every possible pattern during this time: no mood swings during the deepest depression and when euthymic, improvement beginning in the evening with morning lows, relapse beginning in the evening with morning well-being. From Wirz-Justice and Van den Hoofdakker [20], with permission.

use of light therapy for affective disorders *independent of diagnostic subgroup* [23–25, 27, 32].

The potential scope for light therapy extends far beyond narrowly defined major depressive and bipolar disorders. Table 4 lists established and exploratory applications that are showing promise.

1.9 What Is Chronotherapeutics?

Chronotherapeutics encompasses a set of treatments arising from research in chronobiology (light therapy) and from astutely following up clinical observations (sleep deprivation). Psychiatric chronotherapeutics can be defined as controlled exposure to environmental stimuli that act on biological rhythms in order to achieve therapeutic effects in the treatment of psychiatric conditions [21]. The term is broad, although our Manual focuses on affective disorders.

The pineal hormone melatonin, administered as a pill, can, like light, synchronise circadian rhythms and induce sleep [42], and has proved to be very useful for the sleep-wake cycle disorders in persons with visual impairment [43]. Melatonin does not appear to have any major effects on mood by itself.

The major importance of light or melatonin, or both in combination, lies in their zeitgeber characteristics, i.e. their capacity to synchronise or phase shift rhythms. Rhythmic stability appears to be crucial for stable and euthymic mood state [44]. *Internal synchronisation* means appropriate timing between core body rhythms such as cortisol, temperature, and sleep; *external synchronisation* means the appropriate timing of these rhythms with respect to the day-night cycle. As a corollary, one can have internal desynchronisation, when the sleep-wake cycle is no longer correctly in phase with the other core body rhythms, and external desynchronisation, when the inner rhythms are out of phase with the day-night cycle. Two obvious examples of the latter are when we move ourselves into another time zone – either by flying there, so that the inner rhythms have to adapt to a new day-night cycle, or by shift work, where the light-dark cycle remains constant, but we have adopted a different, and often changing, relationship to it.

We think that depression reflects a kind of internal desynchronisation. This hypothesis was first tested when we moved sleep 6 h earlier in a bipolar patient who had responded well to sleep deprivation [45] (fig. 12). If, as postulated, her internal clock was phase advanced with respect to her sleep-wake cycle, perhaps her clinical state might be modified by moving sleep earlier to a more correct phase relationship. It was a remarkable experiment. Over a period of about 3 weeks her mood gradually improved, remained stable for a while, and then gradually got worse again. Daily ratings revealed how a circadian rhythm of mood drifted throughout the wake phase, as though a kind of positive jet lag had been induced (fig. 12). After the relapse into depression, her sleep was phase advanced another 6 h, and a similar 3-week time course of improvement was repeated. This single case study laid the basis for the schematic in figure 10: it was not the deprivation of sleep per se that was antidepressant, but rather being awake at a sleep-sensitive circadian phase.

Internal and external synchronisation are thus important for normal healthy functioning. If internal and external synchronisation are even more important for patients vulnerable to depression, then the emphasis of chronotherapeutics on the role of zeitgebers to stabilise circadian rhythm phase can be well understood [44]. Light and melatonin are the most important zeitgebers, but other synchronising factors, such as the regularity of social schedules and meal times, also play a role. The latter factors have been emphasised in the practice of interpersonal social rhythm therapy (IPSRT, section 14), which has been successful with bipolar patients [46]. Surprisingly, regular exposure to dark periods can attenuate the mood swings of rapid cycling disorder [47, 48]: a preliminary trial of 14 h of 'dark therapy' per night reduced manic symptoms as rapidly as conventional antipsychotics [49].

In summary, circadian rhythm and sleep research has led to non-pharmacologic therapies of depression – light and wake therapy – that can be conveniently applied in everyday practice.

Individual Chronotherapeutic Elements: Light, Wake Therapy and Sleep Phase Advance

'Lethargics are to be laid in the light and exposed to the rays of the sun.' *Aretaeus*, 2nd Century AD

'Preventing sleep may seem cruel but it ameliorates suffering: patients are awakened each time they appear to fall asleep.' *J.A.C. Heinroth*, 1818

Chronotherapeutics for major depression includes three major components:

- Bright light therapy
- Wake therapy (total or partial sleep deprivation)
- Sleep phase advance therapy

Wake and light therapy and sleep phase advance are safe, with a minimal side-effect profile. In combination, they do not interact negatively with ongoing medication (barring photosensitivity in the visible range, e.g. with first-generation neuroleptics). They may also reduce the required duration for hospitalisation in patients with major depression. On one psychiatric unit, the combination of wake therapy (three sessions over a week) with antidepressants allowed discharge three days earlier than with drug treatment alone [Benedetti, unpubl. data]. There was a similar 3-day advantage for depressed patients exposed to more natural light in sunny hospital rooms than those staying in dimmer rooms [50, 51]. Six-month data before and after renovation of an entire psychiatric unit with bright light also yielded an average of 3 days' shorter hospitalisation [52].

2.1 Efficacy of Bright Light Therapy for SAD

Light therapy can be considered the most successful clinical application of chronotherapeutics to date. Light therapy was developed for SAD and over the years the apparatus design modified to provide optimum efficacy. The dosing variables of light therapy are:

- Light intensity
- Duration of exposure
- Time of day of exposure
- Spectral composition
- Field of illumination

The established form of bright light therapy provides broad-spectrum white, UV-filtered, diffuse illumination at an early-morning outdoor daylight level, conventionally 10,000 lx (the level from skylight about 40 min after sunrise). This is the standard that has been tested in controlled clinical trials. At this intensity, 30 min is usually sufficient for treating SAD patients, but flexibility is required to obtain the individual optimum dose. Using lower light intensity (e.g. 2500 lx) at least an hour per day is required. The consensus is that bright light has an antidepressant effect at all times of day greater than placebo (dim) light, but that morning light is superior to evening light. All these factors are summarised by Research Precedent 1. A meta-analysis of controlled trials (fig. 13) provides an overall effect size for light treatment of SAD.

Research Precedent 1
This table reviews the three major double-blind controlled trials of light therapy that established the standards of dosage and timing. In particular, the first two studies of high intensity light and shorter duration show nearly identical results of approximately 55% remission with morning light and 30% with evening light compared with 15% for placebo (a negative ion generator). From Wirz-Justice [53], with permission.

Summary of Remission Rates*

	Remission rate, % (patients)		
	Morning light	Evening light	Placebo
Terman et al.†			
First treatment	54 (25/46)	33 (13/39)	11 (2/19)
Crossover	60 (28/47)	30 (14/47)	ND
Eastman et al.‡			
First treatment	55 (18/33)	28 (9/32)	16 (5/31)
Lewy et al.§			
First treatment	22 (6/27)	4 (1/34)	ND
Crossover	27 (14/51)	4 (2/51)	ND

* Defined as improvement of 50% or more in the score on the Structured Interview Guide for the Hamilton Depression Rating Scale-Seasonal Affective Disorder Version and posttreatment score of 8 or less; recalculated from original data sets. ND = Not done.
† Six-year study; 10,000 lx for 0.5 h, 2 weeks.
‡ Six-year study; 6,000 lx for 1.5 h, 4 weeks.
§ Four-year study; 2,500 lx for 2 h, 2 weeks.

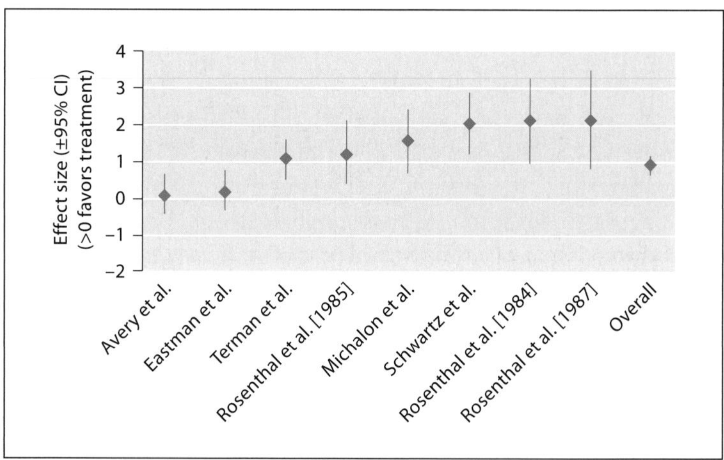

Fig. 13. Effect sizes in studies of treatment of SAD with bright light. From Golden et al. [23], with permission.

2.2 Timing of Bright Light Therapy

As shown above, timing of morning light appears to be important for a better response in SAD patients. The definitions of 'morning' and 'evening' in these studies (and most studies) are according to clock time (external time). However, even better response rates are achieved when individuals are treated with light timed according to circadian phase (internal time). How do we measure internal time? A primary marker is the circadian rhythm of melatonin secretion, which defines the subjective night [10]. More practically, the evening increase in melatonin secretion before bedtime (with samples collected under dim light conditions so as not to inhibit pineal activity) is an accepted standard. Individually determined

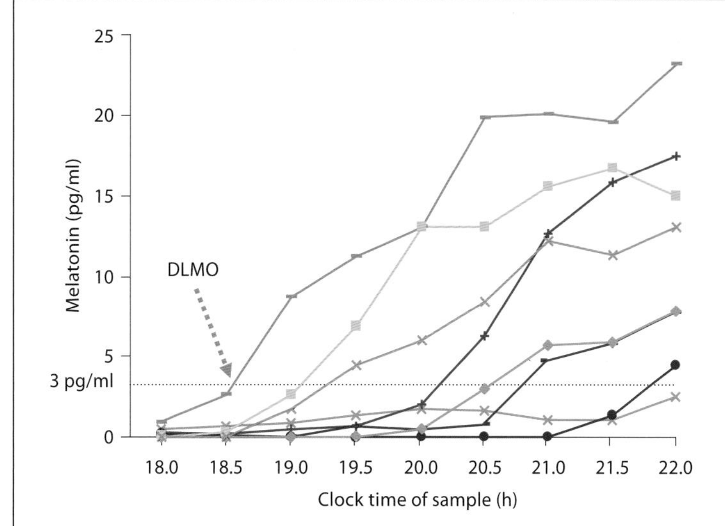

Fig. 14. Evening rise in melatonin secretion in 8 individuals, measured in half-hourly saliva samples with the Bühlmann assay (fig. 16), showing a wide normal range. The threshold for DLMO is taken as 3 pg/ml; an example of DLMO time is shown for the earliest curve. One subject does not attain this threshold by the last saliva sample, i.e. DLMO is later than 10 p.m. [Wirz-Justice, unpubl. data].

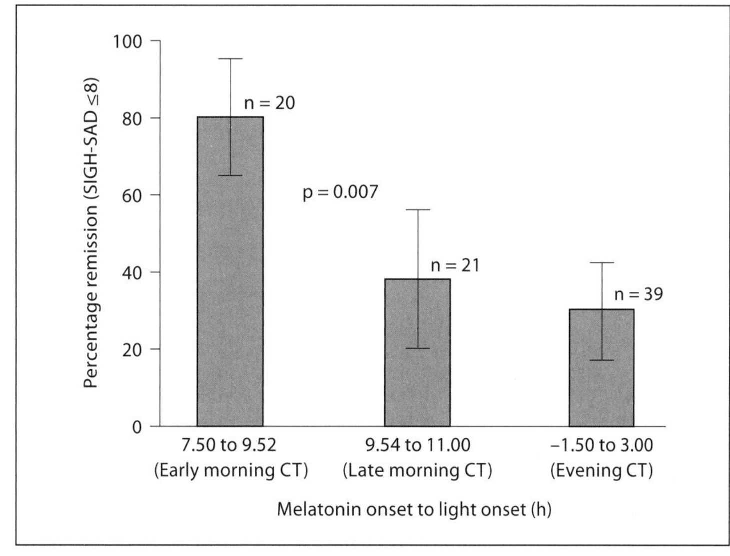

Fig. 15. Remission rate (percentage of subjects ± 95% CI) to 10,000 lx, 30-min light exposure in SAD patients, anchored to the circadian time (CT) of treatment. 0 h CT is specified by the onset of melatonin production. From Terman et al. [27], with permission.

dim light melatonin onset (DLMO) [10] (fig. 14) thus provides an internal reference for timed administration of light therapy. There is a wide range even between normal healthy individuals in their preferences in sleep-wake timing. This range of so-called chronotypes extends from extreme morning 'larks' to late evening 'owls'. The differences in circadian timing in normal healthy individuals are seen when measuring the DLMO (fig. 14): larks may show onset as early as 7 p.m., owls as late at 1 a.m. A wide range is also found in depressed SAD patients. This variability emphasises the need to adjust timing of light therapy to the individual's internal time.

In fact, by forming groups according to timing of light therapy with respect to their internal instead of external time, a doubling of remission rates (80 vs. 40%) with early morning versus late

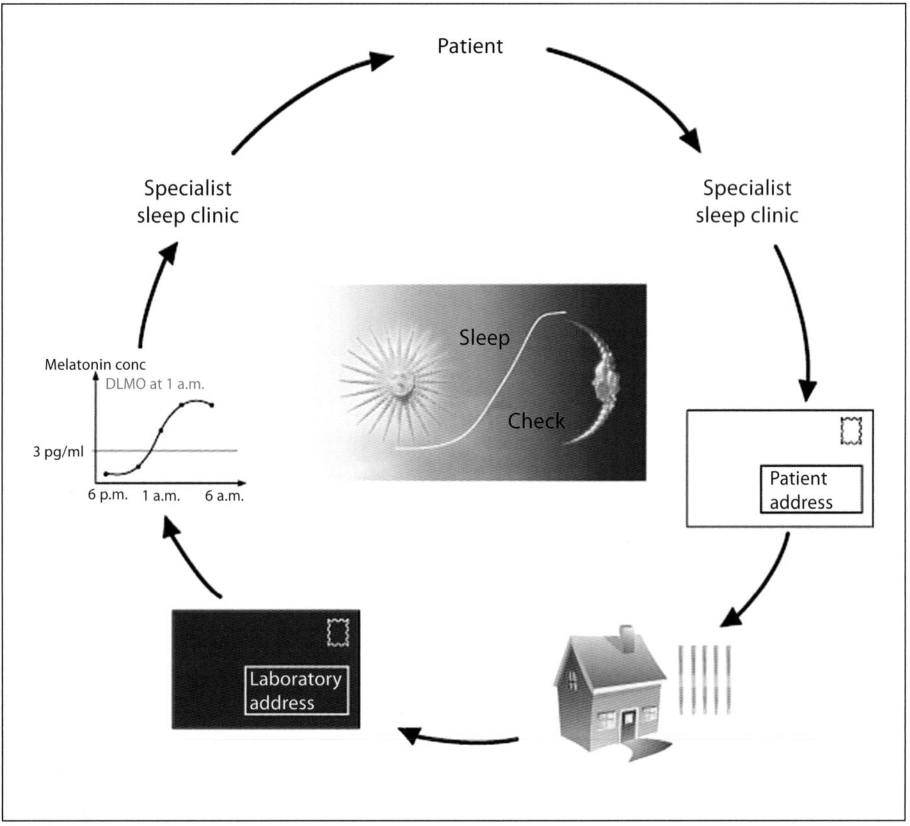

Fig. 16. Method for using the ambulatory saliva collection kit at home for the determination of melatonin onset in sleep disorders. Developed within the www.euclock.org project by Bühlmann Laboratories, Allschwil, Switzerland. The patient collects timed salivary samples in prepared salivettes at home in the evening under dim light conditions. The packet is sent to the lab for assay, and the sleep specialist receives the results with an interpretation of the DLMO found. This information is discussed with the patient and the appropriately timed treatment of the circadian sleep disorder is initiated.

morning treatment was achieved in SAD patients (fig. 15). In terms of circadian rhythms, the greater the phase advance of melatonin onset achieved (up to 2.5 h), the better the response.

Preliminary evidence suggests that this careful timing is also important for non-seasonal major depression, although bipolar patients may respond better to midday light or reduced doses of morning light [55, 56].

In order to improve the diagnosis and therapy of circadian rhythm disturbances, there is now a kit for measuring melatonin rhythms non-invasively in saliva [57] (fig. 16). This has been developed primarily for ambulatory patients in sleep medicine clinics, where the diagnosis of Advanced or Delayed Sleep Phase Disorder can be confirmed by measuring melatonin timing. It would also provide an objective measure of the circadian rhythm disturbance in depressed patients.

Direct measurement of the melatonin rhythm is not always practicable and the clinician may need an on-the-spot assessment. Therefore, a rea-

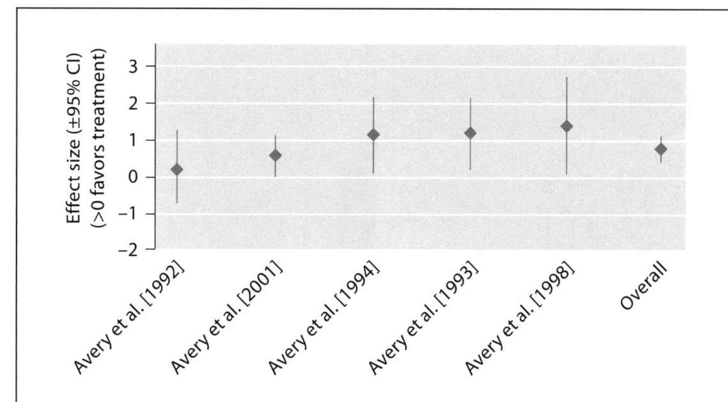

Fig. 17. Effect sizes in studies of treatment of SAD with dawn simulation. From Golden et al. [23], with permission.

sonable estimate of internal body clock time without directly measuring the melatonin rhythm would be useful. A good correlation has been found between an individual's chronotype, based on the total score from the Horne-Östberg Morningness-Eveningness Questionnaire [58] (MEQ, appendix 1) score and DLMO. This has provided an algorithm for timing light treatment, which will be detailed in section 4.2.

2.3 Dawn (and Dusk) Simulation Therapy

One drawback of bright light therapy is the required daily time commitment. By contrast, dawn simulation is presented during the last period of the patient's sleep episode, with a relatively dim signal gradually rising over 90 min or longer from about 0.001 lx (starlight) to approximately 300 lx (sunrise under tree shade). As with bright light therapy, there is an antidepressant response and normalisation of hypersomnic and abnormal sleep patterns.

A large controlled study of SAD compared 3 weeks of treatment with bright light upon habitual wake-up time or dawn simulation gauged against a low-density negative air ion placebo. Both light conditions were superior to placebo and showed comparable efficacy [59]. A summary of earlier results from the University of Washington, entered into a meta-analysis, is shown in figure 17.

In distinction from dawn simulation, dusk simulation at bedtime may help to delay the circadian clock. The combination of dusk and dawn may be useful for stabilising the daily sleep-wake cycle and enhancing sleep continuity [39]. Clinically, the dusk signal is perceived by patients as hypnotic.

Dawn and dusk simulation (DDS) therapy provides a major departure from standard bright light therapy in the following ways:

- DDS therapy is used while in bed, during normal sleep hours. By contrast, bright light therapy is used during waking hours.
- DDS therapy presents gradually changing light levels to mimic outdoor dawn and dusk transitions (when the sun is below the horizon). The maximum required light intensity is around 300 lx. By contrast, bright light therapy presents constant light at supra-sunrise levels (e.g. 10,000 lx).
- DDS is a more practical, 'automatic' treatment in that it hardly requires the user's attention, and most of the signal is presented while the user is asleep. By contrast, bright light therapy requires scheduling waking hours for treatment.

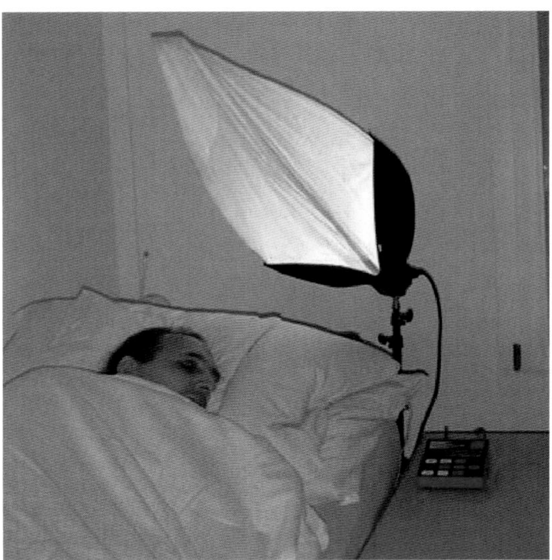

Fig. 18. A dawn-dusk delivery system over the bed with control console at the bedside (Center for Environmental Therapeutics).

Although dawn simulation therapy appears advantageous, there have been far fewer clinical trials using this method. Most tests have used a dawn signal alone, without the dusk signal, with overall results similar to that of bright light therapy: increased ease of awakening, with more alertness and energy, and an antidepressant effect. Case studies using a combination of dusk and dawn signals are very promising [39]. The dusk twilight fade is scheduled around bedtime, and the dawn reaches its peak around wake-up time. People who have had difficulty falling asleep report smoother sleep onset in the presence of a dusk fade.

Apparatus for DDS delivery varies widely in design and adherence to the outdoor naturalistic pattern. Choice of lamp and fixture is important, with the goal of bathing the sleeping area in a diffuse light signal that will reach the eyes as sleeping posture varies (example of a prototype in fig. 18).

The initial demonstration of DDS therapy in a case series in the late 1980s [60] showed that:

- The dim dawn signal served to cut short the body's production of melatonin in the morning hours, which probably contributed to the increased ease of awakening.
- After a week of daily home exposure to a naturalistic dawn set for early May (but delivered in midwinter, see fig. 4), the circadian rhythm of melatonin production shifted to an earlier hour. Thus, the dawn simulation had a physiological effect of mimicking earlier melatonin rhythms in spring.

The authors concluded that 'twilight exposure appears able to promote circadian phase adjustments, morning melatonin suppression, regularised sleep patterns, and antidepressant responses. This represents the first indication in humans of physiological and/or behavioural sensitivity to such light signals' [60]. Underscoring the logic of DDS versus bright light therapy, the authors continued, 'We hypothesise that non-modulated bright light constitutes a supernormal stimulus (that is, a stimulus with higher intensity than required under natural conditions). The eyes may be primed at twilight hours for reception of changing intensities of low-level light' [60].

In a recent randomised, controlled, parallel-group study of 58 patients with SAD, dawn simulation produced a mean DLMO phase advance of 0.58 h, morning bright light therapy produced an advance of 0.70 h, and a low-density negative air ion placebo produced a delay of 0.19 h [$p < 0.001$, Terman and Terman, unpubl. data]. Neither the phase shift nor the antidepressant effect differed between active conditions, while there was negligible clinical improvement on placebo, accompanied by a small phase delay of DLMO [89].

In controlled laboratory studies of healthy young subjects, a single dawn pulse was able to phase advance melatonin onset the next night, demonstrating an acute physiologic effect of the signal [61]. With repeated dawn presentations, the signal forestalled the natural delay drift of the circadian system [62].

The effectiveness of dawn simulation may depend on the presentation of diffuse, broad-field illumination that reaches the sleeper in varying postures. Such results have not been demonstrated for commercial 'light alarm clocks'. Several inexpensive devices have been marketed, cloning the DDS concept, but with rapid dawn ramps (far faster than natural dawns) and restricted fields of illumination. These mass-market products have not yet received adequate clinical evaluation.

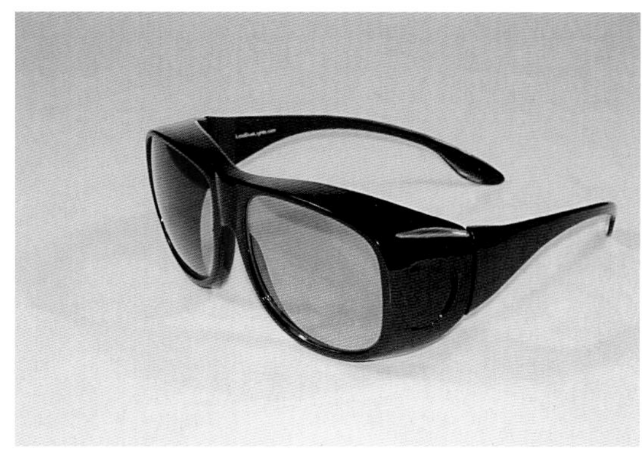

Fig. 19. Amber filters in glasses worn to filter short-wavelength light <535 nm (Center for Environmental Therapeutics).

2.4 Efficacy of Bright Light Therapy for Non-Seasonal Depression

Beyond its established application for SAD, light therapy for non-seasonal depression appears both safe and effective. In a comparison of the relative benefit of light therapy to placebo controls, 1 week of treatment produced as much improvement as 4–16 weeks of treatment with antidepressant drugs [31]. Few of the early light studies in non-seasonal depression have been of sufficient duration to compare with treatment-as-usual. Light treatment in patients with chronic major depression achieved a surprising remission rate of 50% compared with a placebo (low-density negative air ionisation) [41].

2.5 Dark Therapy

In rapid cycling bipolar disorder the recurrent pattern can be halted immediately by extending darkness (or rest, or sleep), which is an impressive result for these therapy-resistant patients [47, 48]. Furthermore, manic symptoms in bipolar patients can be diminished under extended darkness (not merely rest or sleep) with improvement as rapid as with conventional antipsychotic treatment [49]. Thus, we see parallels in light's action on depression and darkness for mania. Since keeping manic patients for a long period in darkness is infeasible in clinical practice, a similar result can be achieved with eyeglasses that specifically filter out the circadian-sensitive blue wavelengths. A pilot study of these amber-coloured glasses (example in fig. 19) showed improvement in 50% of bipolar patients with sleep onset insomnia [63].

A physiological consequence of short wavelength filtering is the protection of endogenous pineal melatonin production without light-induced suppression. This may help stabilise day-to-day sleep-wake cycles and consequent mood lability.

2.6 Wake Therapy

The slow response to most antidepressants is the biggest problem for psychiatrists and their patients. In remarkable contrast is the improvement, within hours, of staying awake all night. Response to a single wake therapy session occurs

Research Precedent 2
Time course of depression self-ratings before, during and after a total sleep deprivation and recovery sleep. Controls maintain low depression ratings, patients either respond (the day after) or not. Redrawn from Gerner et al. [64], with permission.

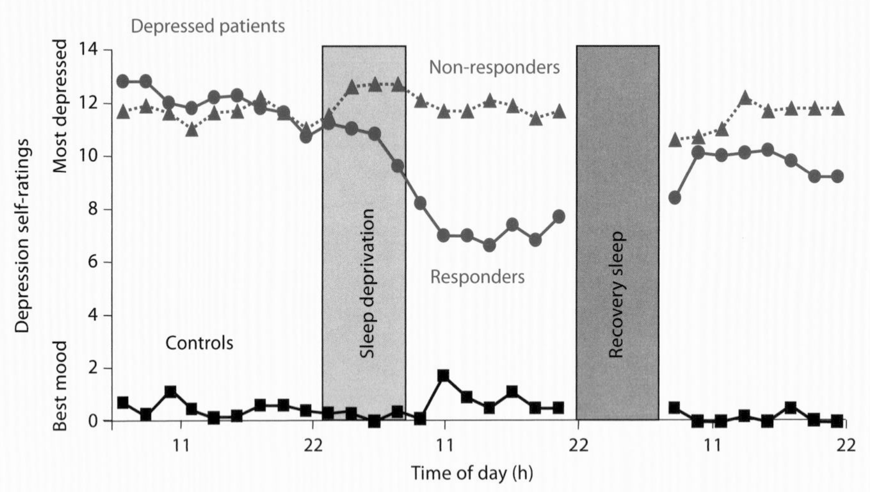

in approximately 60% of patients with major depression, across all diagnostic subgroups [20]. Research Precedent 2 demonstrates this rapid time course in a group of depressed patients.

Because relapse usually follows recovery sleep (or even short daytime naps), this unusual treatment has not caught on except in German-speaking countries where it was first described. It has taken a new generation of researchers to be inventive, and after attaining fast response with one or more nights of wake therapy, adding various treatments to hold that response. As an attempt to lessen the stress of an entire night's sleep deprivation, total versus partial sleep deprivation has been compared, as well as the first half of the night being awake versus the second half of the night [20]. In general, the consensus is that being awake in the second half of the night is crucial for the antidepressant response (fig. 10).

2.7 Phase Advance of the Sleep-Wake Cycle

A crucial experiment that shifted the timing of the sleep-wake cycle 6 h earlier demonstrated that being awake during the second half of the night was critical for antidepressant response rather than the sleep deprivation per se [45]. The improvement occurred more slowly (over 3 days) than the acute single total sleep deprivation, but lasted longer (3 weeks). The analogy with jet-lag supported the idea that it was important to realign abnormal phase relationships.

Although challenging to carry out the sleep scheduling procedure on an inpatient unit, it was theoretically important, and led to further studies comparing sleep phase advance with sleep phase delay following a single total sleep deprivation [65]. Shorter and more practical versions of sleep phase advance therapy have now been implemented [66, 67] (Research Precedents 3 and 4).

Research Precedent 3
Bipolar depressed patients carried out sleep deprivation followed by a 3-day phase advance of the sleep period (day 1, bedtime from 5 p.m. to 12 a.m.; day 2, 7 p.m. to 2 a.m.; day 3, 9 p.m. to 4 a.m.). This was sufficient to prevent relapse for at least 5 days, the response being greater in lithium-treated patients (redrawn from Benedetti et al. [66], with permission).

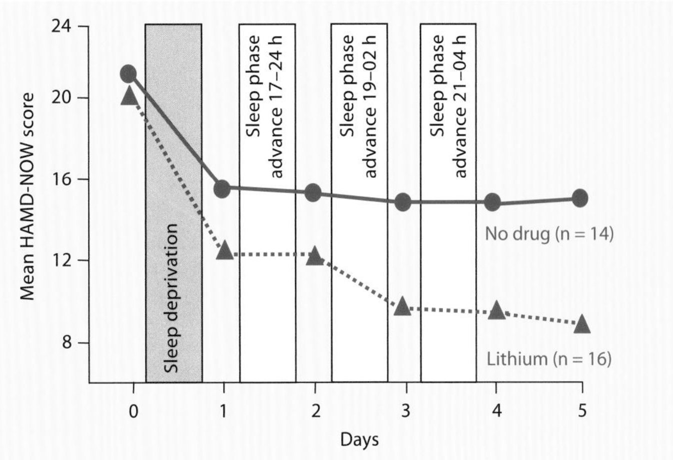

Research Precedent 4
Unipolar depressed patients who responded to sleep deprivation carried out a 3-day phase advance of the sleep period (day 1, bedtime from 5 p.m. to 12 a.m.; day 2, 7 p.m. to 2 a.m.; day 3, 9 p.m. to 4 a.m.). This was sufficient to prevent relapse for at least 6 days (redrawn from Voderholzer et al. [67], with permission).

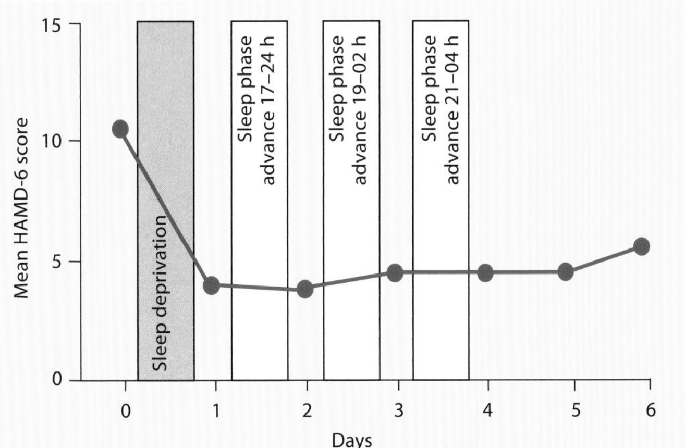

In particular, following a total night's sleep deprivation, there is little difficulty in asking a tired but no longer depressed patient to go to bed at 5 or 6 p.m. In the above research examples, the sleep period was shifted to 7 p.m. on the second night, and 9 p.m. on the third night. This 3-day phase-advance option has recently been used together with a single sleep deprivation and 3 days light therapy to improve bipolar depressed patients on medication more rapidly than medication alone [68].

2.8 Negative Air Ionisation

Negative air ionisation is not directly within the purlieu of chronobiology, but as a novel non-invasive non-pharmacologic intervention, it has potential interest as an adjuvant comparable to chronotherapeutics. There is some older literature suggesting positive effects on mood. The mechanisms of action are still unknown, although both serotonergic stimulation and enhanced blood oxygenation have been hypothesised. The air circulation outdoors varies greatly in negative ion content (higher in humid, vegetated environments and at the seashore; lower in urban environments and heated or air-conditioned interiors).

The apparatus was first used in a number of controlled light therapy trials as a non-pharmaceutical inert placebo. The apparatus did not emit negative ions (which in any case are imperceptible) in spite of being turned on with a fan noise and indicator light. A controlled trial for treatment of SAD used low-density negative ions as the placebo, but had also a group receiving high-density negative ions [69]. The antidepressant response, which appeared after 2 weeks of 30 min exposure sessions every morning, was specific to the high dose condition. In a second study, patients received high- or low-density negative air ionisation for 90 min before habitual wake-up time [59]. After 2 weeks, a therapeutic effect was again obtained only under the high dose condition. The ionisation trials were folded into parallel group protocols including light therapy, with similar improvement. In follow-up, some patients responded to ions but not to light, and vice versa. This suggests that the mechanism of action of the ion effect does not necessarily involve circadian timing. Indeed, the mean DLMO phase advance to high-density ions (0.03 h) was not significantly different from the phase delay to low-density ions (0.19 h) [Terman and Terman, unpublished data].

Since we are interested in developing non-invasive environmental therapeutics, not only chronobiologically based methods, negative air ionisation is an intriguing new treatment possibility that requires further study.

Integrative Chronotherapeutics: Combinations of Light, Wake Therapy and Sleep Phase Advance

This Manual focuses on several combination strategies that induce and maintain rapid antidepressant response.

3.1 A Note on Diagnostic Differences

Before going into detail, some clear statements should be made about the unipolar/bipolar dichotomy and the use of long-term prophylactic medication. Patients affected by major depressive disorder or by bipolar disorder suffer from recurrent episodes of mood illness throughout their lifetime, and frequency and severity are the major determinants of the disabling effects of the illness. In both conditions depression plays the major role, and bipolar patients are expected to suffer from depression three times more than from mania, and are found to be depressed in 30% of random interviews [70]. In both conditions, the prevention of recurrence, and of depression in particular, is the major goal of long-term therapy and has the highest impact on quality of life.

Following current guidelines, the mainstay for preventive interventions is long-term pharmacologic treatment, but neurochemical strategies differ between the two disorders. Patients affected by unipolar depression are usually treated with antidepressant drugs, and patients affected by bipolar disorder are treated with lithium salts and other mood stabilisers in order to avoid the mania-inducing effect of antidepressants. Nevertheless, the acute pharmacologic treatment of bipolar depression with an antidepressant leads to a need of prolonged treatment, because drugs cannot be stopped before six months for risk of relapse [71].

Integrative chronotherapeutics provides techniques for the acute treatment of depression, which can be added to pharmacologic treatment-as-usual of unipolar and bipolar depression. The aim is to speed up response at the start of the depressive episode, since antidepressants show long latency of action. In addition, chronotherapeutics reduces reliance on antidepressants because of its independent action. Longer-term chronotherapeutics may be useful during prolonged drug treatment, which poses a risk of manic relapse.

'Pure' switching between depression and mania is not the only psychopathological condition that affects bipolar patients, who may also experience mixed states in which symptoms pertaining to both conditions occur simultaneously. The current nosological status of these mood episodes relies more on classical medical reasoning: mixed states show a good response to antimanic treatment, with particular sensitivity to antiepileptic mood stabilisers.

It is thus a clinical error to administer antidepressant drugs during a mixed state. Similarly, it may be risky to administer light therapy, which might exacerbate mood swings; likewise, sleep deprivation, which might transform the mixed state into frank mania.

The diagnosis of mixed states is anything but easy, and relies on both the empathic abilities of the clinician – which are needed, for example, to differentiate the usual irritability seen in adolescent 'pure' depression from the irritability in an adult mixed state – and the concurrent use of structured or semi-structured instruments for both depression and mania (e.g. appendix 7) for a comprehensive evaluation. In deciding when and how to use chronotherapeutics, the clinician needs to distinguish between simple depression and a mixed state, recognising that circadian phase shifts may exacerbate an underlying manic component.

In conclusion, we emphasise that light therapy, sleep deprivation and sleep phase advance are potent neurobiological interventions that can worsen underlying manic states and, indeed, trigger rapid cycling (Case Study 1).

Case Study 1
Rapid Cycling after Too Fast a Sleep Phase Advance

A bipolar patient who underwent the first 6-hour phase advance [45] improved after shifting sleep to 5 p.m. After relapse 3 weeks later sleep was again phase advanced 6 h to 11 a.m., with improvement lasting another 3 weeks. We then tried a prophylactic strategy by phase advancing sleep 6 h before the next anticipated relapse. The patient switched into a rapid cycling pattern of 3 days severe depression and 1 day mania that could no longer be controlled by rescheduling the sleep-wake cycle. Although the first and second phase advance regimens were extremely successful, the third attempt, with too rapid an advance, plunged the patient into rapid cycling. The potency of these interventions, whether productive or deleterious, was obvious [Wehr and Wirz-Justice].

Some bipolar patients are extremely sensitive to light therapy, and early morning treatment may induce or exacerbate mixed states [55, 56]. Midday light exposure, in contrast, can work to improve mood without inducing agitation. Case Study 2 illustrates this point.

Case Study 2
Bipolar Depression and Light Therapy

A bipolar patient in Novosibirsk had experienced her first depressed and hypomanic phases at age 22. Depressions significantly outnumbered and lasted longer than hypomanic episodes. She experienced rapid (within 1 day) switches from depression to hypomania (which lasted less than 1 month). Her depression was characterised by atypical features, but anxiety often prevailed in affect. Although not reaching the criteria for SAD, she entered a light treatment trial at age 29. After morning light (8–10 a.m., 2,500 lx, for 1 week), she experienced clear activation and improved mood, but anxiety, irritability, and a feeling of dissatisfaction also increased. The negative effect was brief, but with repeated daily light exposures became more prominent. When switched to afternoon light (4–6 p.m.), she felt better than after morning light, with no mixed state. Since 1991, the patient has regularly used light therapy at home for 15–20 min in the afternoon [Danilenko and Putilov].

3.2 Bright Light Augmentation of Antidepressant Drug Treatment

The accumulated data on light therapy for both SAD and non-seasonal depression support its broader application in psychiatric clinical practice, whether or not as monotherapy. Clinicians should consider adjunctive light therapy when there is delayed or only partial response to antidepressants. Emerging data suggest that light therapy be used as a first-line treatment given together with the chosen antidepressant. Existing data suggest that the net benefit from adjunctive bright light to SSRIs or TCAs is of the order of 30%. Light therapy offers an important additional step toward reducing residual symptoms and lowering the probability of relapse – at low cost and with minimal side effects.

Combination of light with drugs accelerates improvement relative to drugs alone, a method already in widespread use with European inpatients. Green light (400 lx, 30 min) added to citalopram treatment in patients with major depressive disorder and bipolar disorder hastened and potentiated the antidepressant effect [33] (Research Precedent 5). A large Danish outpatient trial for patients with non-seasonal depression on

Research Precedent 5
A randomised controlled study of SSRI plus adjuvant green light versus placebo (deactivated negative ion generator) in patients with non-seasonal major depression, showing significantly more rapid improvement and greater symptom reduction with light (redrawn from [33], with permission).

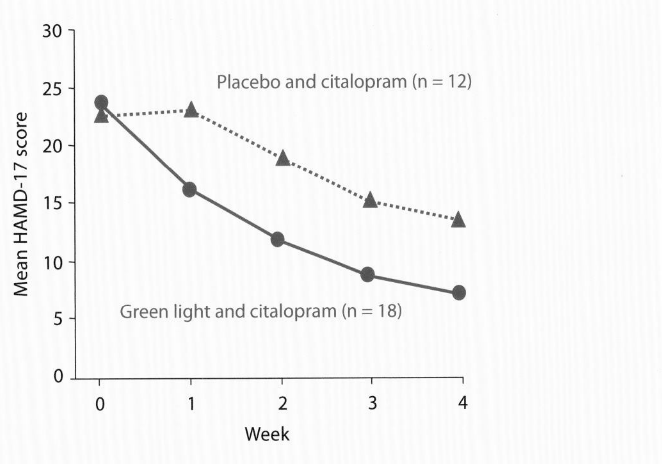

Research Precedent 6
A randomised controlled study of SSRI plus adjuvant bright light versus dim red light in patients with non-seasonal major depression, showing significantly more rapid improvement and greater symptom reduction with bright light (redrawn from [34], with permission).

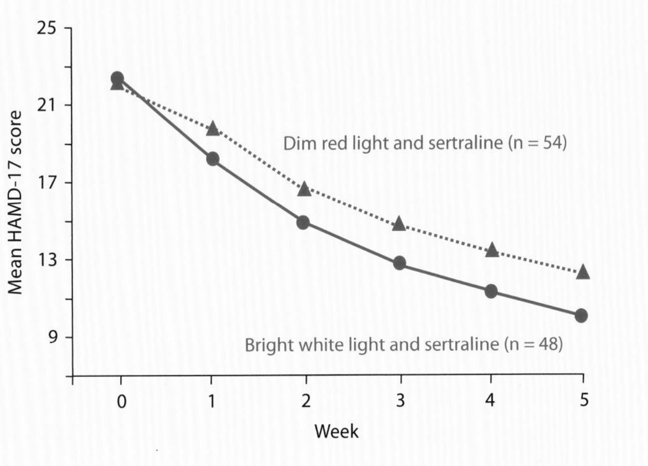

sertraline treatment (n = 102) found that remission rate and speed of improvement were greater under the active white light condition (10,000 lx, 60 min) than placebo red light (50 lx, 30 min) [34] (Research Precedent 6). Discontinuation of light therapy resulted in relapse (similar to findings on withdrawal of antidepressants). Another large study of patients with SAD (n = 282) found that the relapse after discontinuation of light therapy could be prevented by citalopram [72].

Even chronically depressed patients, whose illness had lasted at least 2 years, responded to adjunctive light therapy, a finding of great clinical importance [41]. An even more striking application of light therapy for non-seasonal depression is in adjunctive treatment for treatment-resistant depression, as exemplified in Case Study 3. More trials of these combinations are required to establish a solid evidence base, but given the lack of side effects, the ease of application, and the often rapid improvement that had not been attained with antidepressant drugs alone, adding light therapy seems to be widely indicated.

Case Study 3
Treatment-Resistant Chronic Depression and Light Therapy
A 24-year-old single woman in New York with a lifetime history of dysthymia and a history of anorexia and social phobia had suffered from chronic major depression for 6 years. She was unresponsive to multiple drug trials. Treatment with the monoamine oxidase inhibitor tranylcypromine 100 mg induced a full complement of early, middle, and late insomnia. Light therapy at 7 a.m. for 30 min promptly coalesced sleep (11:30 p.m. to 7 a.m.), and within 3 weeks the patient showed complete remission and was discharged. She continued with light + tranylcypromine at home, but was not compliant with light treatment. Whenever she stopped using the light, she would experience relapse within 2 days. On resumption of the light, she would feel improvement within 2 days and complete remission in 4 days. Although light alone might have maintained her improvement, with such a serious chronic depression it is difficult for psychiatrists to withdraw the drug and rely on light monotherapy [32].

3.3 Wake Therapy Added to Medication

The earliest observations in the 1970s of rapid clinical remission under wake therapy prompted the question whether wake therapy might potentiate the response to medication [20]. Rather than increasing antidepressant dosage for non-responders, adding wake therapy can trigger improvement.

Case Study 4 demonstrates that wake therapy can alleviate depression in lithium-treated bipolar patients.

Case Study 4
Bipolar Depression and Wake Therapy
A 51-year-old woman with difficult-to-treat bipolar 1 disorder was hospitalised in the Ospedale San Raffaele in Milano during a depressive episode that had lasted 8 months. After five mood episodes and three forced hospitalisations in 2 years, with so many disappointing therapeutic failures, the patient and her family became very pessimistic about psychiatry in general, so it was no surprise that they were skeptical about trying the chronotherapeutic approach. Upon admission, all medication was stopped, except for lithium, which was increased. She underwent three consecutive cycles of total sleep deprivation, each followed by a recovery night sleep. However, after the first wake therapy she experienced rapid and complete amelioration of the depressive syndrome leading to perceived euthymia in the early morning. The first recovery sleep was followed by a partial but definite depressive relapse. The second wake therapy led again to perceived euthymia, without relapse after recovery sleep, a benefit sustained after the third wake therapy. Euthymia persisted over the following days and the patient was discharged. High plasma lithium levels were maintained for 6 months, and then reduced to a target level of 0.75 mEq/l. Nine years later, the patient is still euthymic. She still takes lithium, which also prevents the moderate seasonal mood fluctuations which had recurred over her lifetime. Her brother, who suffered from severe bipolar disorder, also showed a good response to wake therapy for depression and dark therapy for mania [Benedetti].

Table 5. Medications that have been used with wake therapy

Lithium	Amitriptyline	Desipramine
Clomipramine	Nortriptyline	Amineptine
Fluoxetine	Sertraline	Paroxetine
Fluvoxamine	Duloxetine	Maprotiline
Pindolol		

Wake therapy appears to be synergistic with antidepressant drugs that potentiate monoaminergic neurotransmission, and lithium salts. Many trials have used both TCAs and newer antidepressants: sleep deprivation hastens and potentiates the response to antidepressants acting on all neurotransmitter target systems (serotonin, noradrenaline, dopamine), and mixed drugs (table 5). The only negative finding comes from a single study combining wake therapy with the antidopaminergic, sedative substance, trimipramine [73]. Indeed, patients do not respond well to sleep deprivation when on neuroleptics (dopamine antagonists).

Research Precedent 7
Responders to partial sleep deprivation in the second half of the night were given dim light (placebo) or bright light for a week. Patients on bright light did not relapse (redrawn from [74], with permisson).

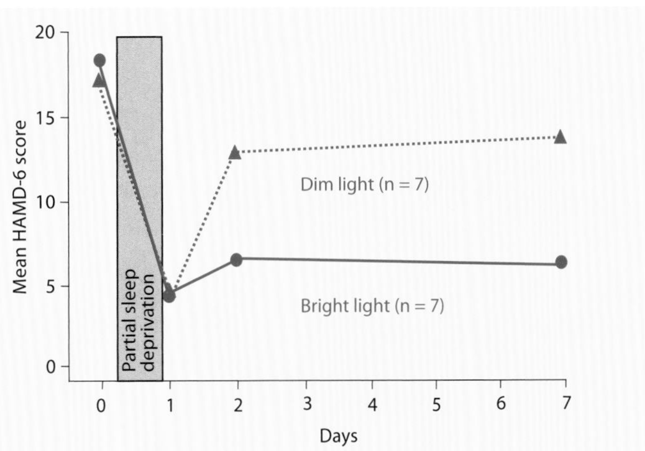

Ideally, wake therapy is administered when beginning medication, so rapid mood improvement occurs during the latency of action of antidepressants. From a practical point of view, both the patient and physician can expect substantial improvement during the most painful days when adequate medication has been prescribed, but has not taken effect. Moreover, the short-term response to wake therapy predicts long-term response to drug [20]. Even during the latency of action, medication can sustain the antidepressant effect of wake therapy, and prevent the usual relapse after recovery sleep.

3.4 Wake and Light Therapy Added to Antidepressant Drugs or Mood Stabilisers

In an expanded protocol, medicated patients with non-seasonal unipolar depression received light therapy and a single session of late-night wake therapy at the start of treatment [74]. There was marked improvement in one day and benefit over a dim light control within one week (Research Precedent 7). In Milano, this model has been extended to general inpatient use, guided by successful treatment studies of non-seasonal major depression (in conjunction with citalopram) and bipolar disorder (in conjunction with lithium), both of which showed large benefits attributable to morning light therapy.

Case Study 5 demonstrates how a colleague who had never administered sleep deprivation became convinced of its efficacy.

Case Study 5
Very First Experience of Combined Wake and Light Therapy in a Copenhagen Hospital
Mrs. K was 65 years old and had a 30-year-long history of bipolar illness. Her depressive episodes often lasted more than 3/4 of a year and did not much improve on antidepressant treatment, whereas her manic periods responded well to low doses of neuroleptics. In her previous depressive episode, which had lasted for 2 months without any sign of improvement, she had heard from her doctor of the possibility of carrying out wake therapy. She was admitted to an open unit, diagnosed with Major Depression with a score of 18 on the Hamilton Depression rating scale. Her medication was left unchanged. She did not have any problem staying up all night. In the morning, her Hamilton score was reduced to 2. After a normal night of sleep she performed two more total sleep deprivations interspersed with a normal night's sleep. During the early morning of the sleep deprivations she received 30 min of light therapy (10,000 lx), which was repeated later that morning. Her Hamilton score remained below 3 and she was discharged after 5 days. At home, she continued daily light treatment and was able to avoid sleep-

ing during the day. She filled in a self-evaluation questionnaire for depression for the subsequent 28 days, without any sign of relapse [Martiny].

Large-scale trials in Europe strongly support the implementation of adjunctive light and wake therapy for treatment of non-seasonal major depression, with the prospect of reduced duration of hospitalisation. Combined wake and light therapy improved the acute response in patients with bipolar 1 disorder treated with antidepressants and lithium salts: 44% of drug-resistant patients responded, and 70% with no previous history of drug-resistance improved [75]. Importantly, a 9-month follow-up showed that 57% of non-resistant responders (but only 17% of drug-resistant responders) remained euthymic [75]. This is the first study to document long-term remission rate enhanced by chronotherapeutics. Two new unpublished studies have found that a single week of chronotherapeutic augmentation not only accelerated and potentiated clinical response, but maintained it for at least 7 weeks or 28 weeks follow-up. Case Study 6 documents the response of a representative patient in the latter study.

Case Study 6
Unipolar Depression with Wake Therapy, Light and Duloxetine

Mr. L, 55 years old, had experienced two previous depressive episodes in 2002 and 2004, probably both stress induced. Each episode required long-term sick leave, but he had not been really well since 2004, in spite of antidepressant drug treatment. He developed a disturbed sleep pattern with sleep onset delayed to 2–3 a.m. and daytime naps of long duration. He was referred to a chronotherapeutic study in August 2008, with a HAMD score of 20 in spite of antidepressant treatment with duloxetine 60 mg since that spring. On admission, his medication was left unchanged. He carried out three total sleep deprivations, each separated by a phase advanced recovery sleep from 7 p.m. to 7 a.m. The wake therapy was done at home with the help of his fiancée. In the morning after sleep deprivation, he was treated with 30 min of bright light therapy (10,000 lx) at 7 a.m. (scheduled according to his chronotype score on the Morningness-Eveningness scale). He continued with daily light therapy and was advised to maintain a regular sleep-wake cycle. His HAMD scores declined weekly to 14, 12, 10, 8 and 5 six weeks later. The depression had remitted and sleep had almost normalised [Martiny].

3.5 Wake, Light, and Sleep Phase Advance Therapy

In initial studies, wake therapy was combined with a sleep phase advance. Later, a controlled trial demonstrated the superiority of a phase advance over a phase delay to maintain the wake therapy response [65]. The full, three-part chronotherapeutics combination is just beginning to see application. Three recently completed studies indicate the scope of improvement achieved.

- In bipolar patients, antidepressants were combined with a week-long protocol of a single wake therapy, 3 days light therapy, and 3 days sleep phase advance [68]. The chronotherapeutics group improved significantly faster and with greater symptom reduction than the treatment-as-usual group, and remained better over 7 weeks. Thus, acute chronotherapeutics has a lasting effect above-and-beyond accelerating the improvement to medication.
- In patients with unipolar disorder, duloxetine combined with wake therapy, light therapy, and sleep hygiene – which emphasised the importance of maintaining a stable sleep cycle, not a phase advance per se – was compared with a control group given duloxetine and a daily exercise programme. The chronotherapeutic intervention induced a rapid and sustained response – still found at 28 weeks – superior to the response seen under the exercise regimen [76].

- A third trial combined multiple chronotherapeutic interventions during a four-day hospitalisation of 12 patients with major depression: (a) sleep deprivation during the second half of the night; (b) dawn simulation to support early awakening; (c) medium (green) wavelength light at standard room-light level to maintain wakefulness for the duration of the night; (d) morning bright light therapy, and (e) recovery-sleep phase advance [77]. All patients responded rapidly and were discharged. Antidepressants were not used during the procedure or at home following discharge. There were no dropouts or compliance difficulties, and patient satisfaction was high. All patients remained well at 4 weeks of follow-up. The authors noted that although the intervention may appear complex, it was safe, easy to conduct, and required relatively low-cost technology, thus showing high cost efficiency. As a pilot study, the sample was small, and there was no control group. However, such encouraging results clearly warrant validation in controlled clinical trials.

As an alternative to the structured timing of sleep phase advance therapy, patients at the Ospedale San Raffaele in Milano are offered a sheltered environment where they are encouraged to go to bed as soon as they feel tired the evening after a total sleep deprivation, and to sleep as long as they like. While the objective is to advance sleep onset, sleep duration is not controlled nor early morning awakening enforced. The benefit of spontaneous early sleep onset is achieved, and this strategy may be more clinically feasible than assigned early bedtimes.

3.6 Repeated Wake Therapy

This protocol was originally developed based on: (a) research observations that the effects of a single night of wake are transient, and that repeating the procedure is well tolerated by the patients [20], and (b) a specific research precedent, showing that patients with bipolar disorder often experience the spontaneous occurrence of 48-hour sleep-wake cycles soon before switching out of depression [78].

Consider that this complex and apparently difficult treatment protocol mimics nature in an attempt to reproduce its vis sanatrix naturae in a hospital setting. Remarkably, although the spontaneous occurrence of this circabidian (approximately 48-hour) sleep pattern in bipolar depressed patients usually precedes manic switches, its administration is associated with a risk of manic switches (5–7%) no higher than that observed with common serotoninergic drugs, and is markedly lower than that observed with mixed serotonergic-noradrenergic drugs (12–15%) [79].

Repeated wake therapy on alternate days does not imply severe sleep loss. The alternation with three nights of undisturbed sleep means that the period of sleep-wake cycle is enlarged from the usual 24 h length (nightly sleep) to 48 h (sleeping one night out of every two). Very rarely do patients abort the treatment because of excessive sleepiness. The full treatment usually involves a spontaneous phase advance of sleep onset. Each wake period lasts 36 h. Thus, if the treatment begins at 7 a.m., the patient is allowed to go to bed at 7 p.m. on the following day. If patients take this opportunity they will usually respect the 'wake maintenance zone' – a period in the evening during which it is nearly impossible to fall asleep – going to bed a couple of hours before their habitual bedtime, and sleeping longer and more soundly than usual. In so doing, repeated wake therapy results in a spontaneous phase advance of sleep onset (but not of morning awakening) on the day after [80]. The size of the phase advance varies individually; clinically, it appears that larger advances correlate positively with the final response to treatment.

4

Inpatient Procedures

Chronotherapeutics is not an alternative to treatment-as-usual – concomitant antidepressants can be continued or administered as required. Inpatients may start chronotherapeutics quickly upon hospital admission, or later if initial interventions (drugs, ECT, etc.) fail. Importantly, chronotherapeutics is compatible with standard interventions and can be implemented simultaneously, with the goal of accelerated improvement, minimisation of residual symptoms, and expedited hospital discharge.

The methods have been developed by separate groups over 20 years of clinical trials. In this Manual, we integrate them into an ensemble that will serve even the most difficult cases. Chronotherapeutic combinations are flexible and should be implemented step-by-step according to the patient's response (or non-response). In any given case, a subset of the procedures can be fully effective. The clinician's task is to monitor state changes as the procedures unfold, to determine how much unfolding is necessary. If the depression remits at the first protocol stage, elaboration may not be needed unless there is a subsequent slump or relapse.

We present examples of current practice in several inpatient units, with growing acceptance by once-skeptical psychiatrists. In particular, New York-Presbyterian Hospital has tested light therapy on an inpatient unit for treatment-resistant patients who are undergoing multiple ECTs, with some success. We are not suggesting that light therapy should replace ECT, but the encouraging results signify a remarkable and important role for this simple treatment even in severe, chronic major depression.

In implementing integrative chronotherapeutics, morning light therapy is introduced after the first night of wake therapy. When hospital operations cannot accommodate wake therapy, or when an ECT schedule has priority, light therapy can provide benefit as the single chronotherapeutic intervention. Therefore, chronotherapeutic options usually begin with light therapy for inpatients and outpatients alike. A second step is light combined with a single night's sleep deprivation. A third step includes a three-day sleep phase advance.

Thereafter, the clinician can try individual combinations of the three components, though the evidence base is still nascent for the multiple protocols. The Milano group has a standard procedure of three cycles of wake therapy and recovery sleep, combined with light. Their timing of the sleep phase advance on the nights of recovery sleep is flexible, depending on when the patient is ready for bed. In this section, we build from the simplest intervention to the integrated ensemble in stages that parallel clinical decision-making on the unit.

4.1 Response Assessment and Monitoring

An extended version of the Hamilton Depression Scale (SIGH-ADS, appendix 7) provides a structured interview covering both melancholic and atypical symptoms (self-assessment version, appendix 3). A six-item version of the Hamilton Depression Scale has been used for many years in sleep deprivation trials to document the core depressive symptoms and their rapid improvement, leaving out sleep and weight items that are not applicable in this short-term context (appendix 4).

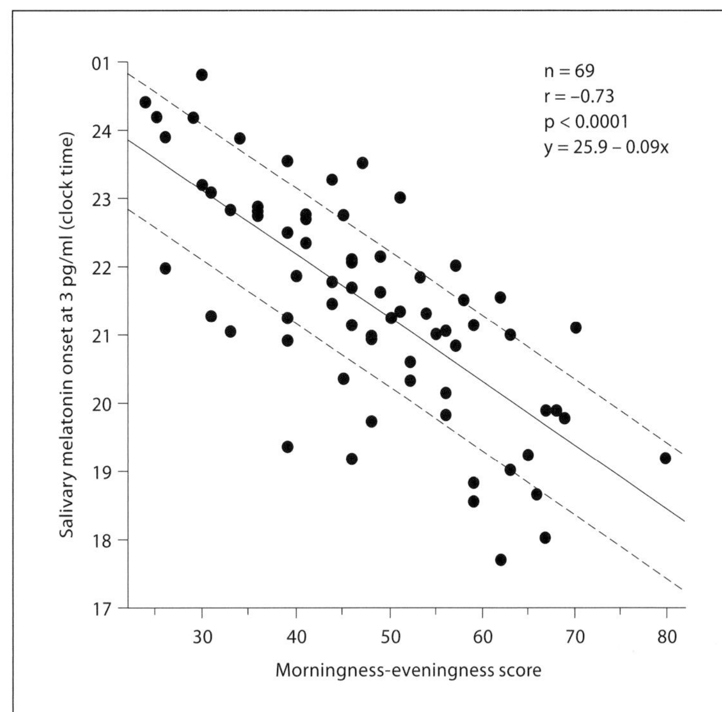

Fig. 20. Correlation of Morningness-Eveningness (MEQ) score and dim light melatonin onset (DLMO) in a group of 69 patients with winter depression. A 10.2-point difference in MEQ score corresponds to a 1-hour difference in DLMO. Solid line = Linear regression; dashed lines = DLMO within 1 h of the MEQ predictor [Terman and Terman, unpubl. data].

Methods

4.2 Light Therapy Timing and Duration

The timing of light therapy is crucial for clinical response in SAD and probably also for non-SAD. Patients – like healthy subjects – vary in their chronotype (e.g. habitual preferred bedtime) by approximately 6 h. Optimum circadian phase advances are achieved with morning light, which should be administered relative to individual internal circadian time, not external clock time. Ideally, this internal clock time is derived from measuring melatonin phase (DLMO) (section 2.2.). Unfortunately, a phase diagnostic based on melatonin assays is not readily available in clinical practice. The melatonin assay remains primarily a research tool, even though such a kit has been developed and is already used in sleep medicine (fig. 16). To provide the clinician a basis to readily specify treatment time, a quick, approximate solution lies in the relation between melatonin onset and the Horne-Östberg Morningness-Eveningness Questionnaire (MEQ; appendix 1) score, which are strongly correlated for unmedicated winter depression patients ($r = -0.73$; fig. 20). Healthy subjects without depression show a similar relationship.

One thus can schedule morning light exposure at individually determined circadian times by estimating the time of melatonin onset from the MEQ score, a strategy that facilitates circadian rhythm phase advances and antidepressant response (fig. 21).

Given the spread of DLMOs around the regression line (fig. 20), there is a risk that light will be scheduled too early, which might lead to premature awakening or counterproductive phase delays. A large clinical trial has shown maximal improvement with light presentation 7.5 h post-DLMO [54]. The MEQ-based recommendation

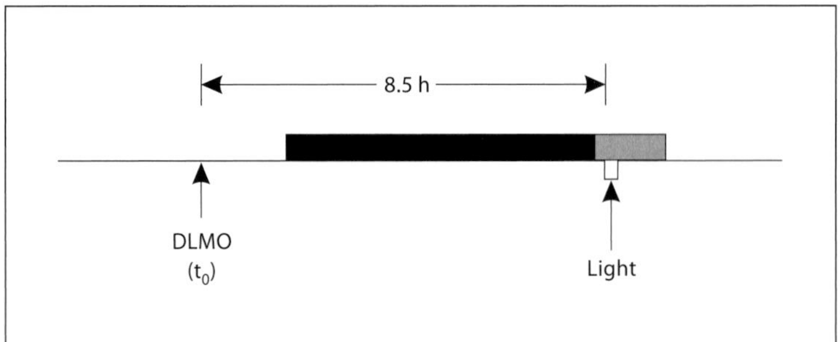

Fig. 21. The relationship between melatonin onset, sleep, and the optimum phase for beginning light therapy. Note that long sleep will require truncation [Terman].

maximises the chance that the patient will receive light in the window of 7.5–9.5 h post-DLMO (fig. 15). With a target time of 8.5 h after DLMO, most patients (44/69, or 64% of the sample) will be captured in this window (±1 h) and 66/69 (96%) will receive light within ±2 h.

An automated, online MEQ is available in English (with PDF downloads also in Danish, English, French, German, Italian, Japanese, Portuguese, Russian and Spanish) at www.cet.org. Calculation of the MEQ score provides the recommended light exposure time for phase advances as well as a coordinated bedtime (table 6).

Hypersomnic patients can initially be scheduled for morning light therapy at the time of habitual awakening and then edged earlier across days toward the target interval. Clinical experience suggests that most of these patients could not sustain earlier awakening without the use of light.

Table 6. Timing of morning light therapy based on MEQ score (beginning of 10,000 lx, 30-min session, approximately 8.5 h after estimated melatonin onset)

MEQ score	Begin light at	MEQ score	Begin light at	MEQ score	Begin light at
16–18	[08:45]	39–41	07:15	62–65	05:45
19–22	[08:30]	42–45	07:00	66–68	05:30
23–26	08:15	46–49	06:45	69–72	05:15
27–30	08:00	50–53	06:30	73–76	05:00
31–34	07:45	54–57	06:15	77–80	[04:45]
35–38	07:30	58–61	06:00	81–84	[04:30]

The algorithm has not been clinically evaluated with scores below 23 and above 76 (from Terman and Terman [81]).

Caveats

The MEQ algorithm to determine internal timing was derived from unmedicated patients with depression. The MEQ score can be distorted by psychotropic medication, comorbid medical disorders, sleep disorders and daily sleep scheduling constraints. Some of the questions cannot be answered by extreme chronotypes whose sleep onset falls outside the normal range (approximately 9 p.m. to 2 a.m.), as in advanced or delayed sleep phase disorder. Such patients may choose the closest 'best answers', resulting in scores of 16–22 or 77–84, when their true chronotype falls outside the scale range. In fact, abnormally advanced sleep phase disorder should be treated with evening, not morning light. In cases where the validity of the MEQ is in question, the timing of light therapy should be based on the habitual sleep-wake cycle.

Benzodiazepines, trazodone and the newer hypnotics mask the sleep-wake cycle without shifting rhythms, and thus perpetuate the internally desynchronised state. In such cases, it is difficult to ascertain the time when subjective night would end in order to appropriately introduce light therapy. The MEQ score can be substantially biased if the patient has become accustomed to sleeping with hypnotics.

In addition, sleep patterns change with clinical state. As one bipolar patient noted: 'Doing the MEQ test made me aware of how much my pattern has changed since I became depressed. Most of my life I was a definite morning type. Now, with the depression and the medication, I have turned into an intermediate type, because my depression lifts in the evening and I feel better at night. Therefore, it was difficult to answer the MEQ questions, because I still feel I am naturally a morning type, but depression has altered my sleep patterns.'

Dosage of light is determined by intensity and exposure duration. In some patients, a 30-min session at 10,000 lx upon awakening will be effective within days, while others will require dose increments. In adjusting dose, the clinician must look for side effects including autonomic hyperactivation, headache and nausea. In bipolar 1 depression, light therapy is never administered without a mood stabiliser, but the clinician must remain alert to manic switches or mixed states. The method has been widely used as monotherapy in outpatients, but is more commonly combined with standard antidepressant medication in both inpatients and outpatients. If a response to light does not emerge within three days, the duration of exposure is gradually increased from 30 to 60 min.

4.3 Exceptions to the Early Morning Light Rule for Bipolar 1 Disorder

The Milano group emphasises careful assessment of mixed states before deciding on therapeutic options (section 3.1.). If a mixed state is apparent in the diagnostic interview, they do not carry out sleep deprivation or light therapy and rely only on mood stabilisers (and the established guidelines for treatment of mixed states). Chronotherapeutics in the case of mixed states with a prevalence of depressive symptoms will almost certainly cause the switch from mixed depression to mixed mania or a frankly manic state.

In a large patient collective of more than 200 patients with bipolar depression (mixed states excluded), a low 5–7% risk of switching into mania with sleep deprivation and light was found, irrespective of treatment with heterogeneous medications [79].

There have also been reports of elicitation of mixed states in bipolar depression or mood lability in rapid cycling bipolar disorder with early morning light exposure, which could be resolved by delaying the morning light therapy session to midday [56]. Caution should be taken with bipolar 1 patients to: (a) diagnose presenting or previous mixed states (with recourse to midday light), and (b) start light exposure duration conservatively at 15 min and increase only cautiously to longer durations. Titration of light dose might be accelerated in closely monitored hospitalised patients.

4.4 Beginning with Light Therapy (± Medication)

Light therapy alone is for patients who refuse sleep deprivation (or clinicians who think it too drastic). Improvement can be rapid, but satisfactory outcome can take several weeks.

We will go through the various combinations assuming a hospitalised patient, for ease of evaluation and monitoring response. The number of days for each step is indicated, but is to be taken as a guide, not a stringent rule, depending on conditions on the unit and the patient's cooperation. Flexibility on the inpatient unit is required, since sleeping on a standardised, enforced unit schedule is counterproductive.

In all cases, the patient is evaluated at admission as a candidate for chronotherapy and the various options are explained. The SIGH-ADS (appendix 7) is administered to assess the depth of depression and the MEQ is completed to assess habitual sleep time and thus chronotype.

The first example (flowchart 1) is for an 8-hour sleeper with MEQ score of 58 (intermediate chronotype). On the evening of hospital admission, the patient is allowed to sleep at his or her habitually preferred time (in this case, 11 p.m. to 7 a.m.).

- Assuming this is a new admission of an unmedicated patient, antidepressants, mood stabilisers, or both are introduced on day 1 or day 2, and acute side effects ascertained before beginning light therapy on day 3. If the patient is taking antidepressant medications, the physicians will assess efficacy and appropriate dosage, and adjust dosing or switch medication upon clinical need. No negative interaction between light therapy and antidepressants has ever been reported, and existing literature shows that the additive effects of light and antidepressant drugs are evident soon after the beginning of the combined treatment. Given a strong response to light therapy, antidepressant (and hypnotic) drug dose may be reduced.
- On day 3 (or sometimes even on day 2), the first light therapy (duration 30 min) is initiated at the MEQ-determined optimum schedule. For this patient with MEQ score of 58, table 6 specifies waking for light administration at 6 a.m., an hour earlier than habitual rise time. The patient is encouraged (but not forced) to remain awake afterwards.
- Bedtime is concomitantly shifted 1 h earlier. Morning light at the designated hour not only truncates the habitual sleep episode, but also shifts the circadian clock earlier. Thus, throughout the course of treatment, in compensation for earlier rising, bedtime is almost always scheduled earlier than before treatment began. The size of advance of wake-up time (starting on day 4) will vary by 0–2 h

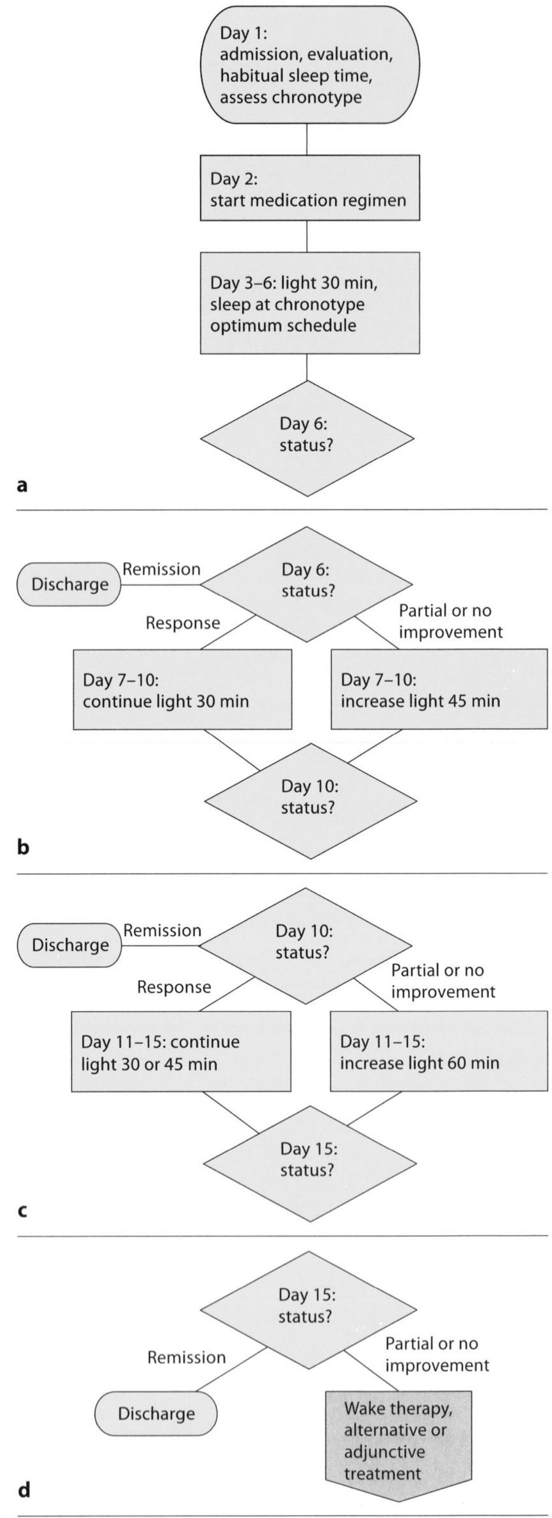

Flowchart 1

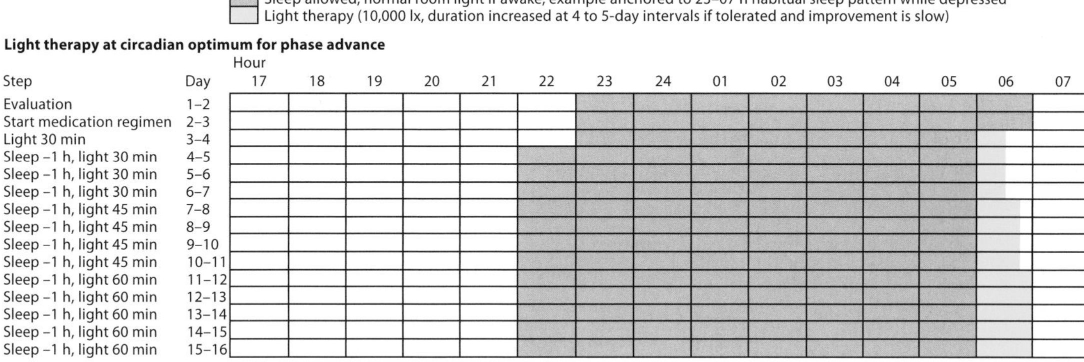

Fig. 22. Timeline encompassing spontaneous sleep while depressed, and the starting time of morning light therapy from the MEQ algorithm. Patients sleeping longer than six hours must truncate morning sleep (by 15 min to 2 h) in order for morning light therapy to provide an optimum phase advance. If necessary, they can compensate with earlier bedtime (in this case, by 1 h).

across patients. Patients with habitually short sleep (in the range of 6 h) will not have to advance wake-up time.

- If the MEQ estimates of 'natural' bedtime and rise time deviate substantially from the patient's reported preferences, both factors need to be taken into account when establishing the light therapy schedule. The compromise solution is midway between MEQ and sleep preference results.
- This schedule is continued until day 6, when a clinical evaluation and the SIGH-ADS score indicate degree of improvement. If remission has occurred, the patient can be discharged with light therapy continued on an outpatient basis at the 30-min dose (appendix 6). If there has been partial or no improvement, light exposure is increased to 45 min for the next 4 days.
- Again, on day 10, clinical evaluation and the SIGH-ADS score indicate whether to discharge, continue with the same light dose, or further increase it to 60 min.
- On day 15, the end of the first phase is reached. If the patient has shown partial improvement or none at all, it is time to add wake therapy (or return to conventional treatment options).

Figure 22 illustrates 2 weeks of treatment, applying the chronobiologic rationale for scheduling light therapy according to sleep timing and duration, using the MEQ algorithm for assuming the patient's melatonin onset.

4.5 Wake Therapy + Light Therapy

The standard course of integrative chronotherapeutics begins with a night of total sleep deprivation followed by continued waking until bedtime the following evening. A single night of sleep deprivation can result in instantaneous remission of depressive symptoms, although the risk of relapse after the next night's sleep is high. Bright light therapy, however, can allay relapse, as can concomitant medication.

As in the previous section, the procedure follows a similar course, illustrated in flowchart 2. After day 6, the procedure follows that of flowchart 1.

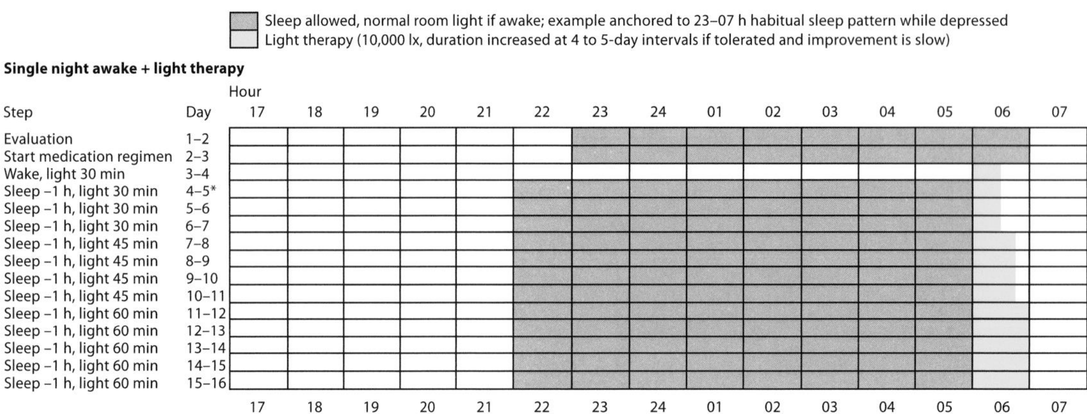

Fig. 23. Timeline for the same patient as in figure 22, encompassing spontaneous sleep while depressed, and the starting time of morning light therapy from the MEQ algorithm, which begins on the morning after sleep deprivation.

- After initial evaluation and commencement of medication, the patient remains awake all night with staff monitoring, starting on the evening of day 3 (section 5 details the management of wake therapy).
- The first light therapy session is scheduled at the MEQ-specified time on the morning after sleep deprivation, day 3.
- The patient remains awake until bedtime on the evening of day 4, which is scheduled 1 h earlier than when treatment began.
- Light therapy duration is incremented by 15 min every 4 days if a full response has not been achieved, as in the previous section.
- Full implementation of integrative chronotherapeutics leads to the initiation of sleep phase advance therapy on day 4 if remission has not occurred after one night of wake therapy.

Using the graphic presentation in figure 23, the schedule for the same patient with a MEQ score of 58 and sleep times from 11 p.m. to 7 a.m. shows the timing of the interventions during the 2 weeks.

So why do we follow up a night awake with light therapy at dawn? Toward the end of the night, the core body temperature rhythm is at its nadir, as are many other functions including mood. This is the time when the circadian system is highly sensitive to light. Timing of light ac-

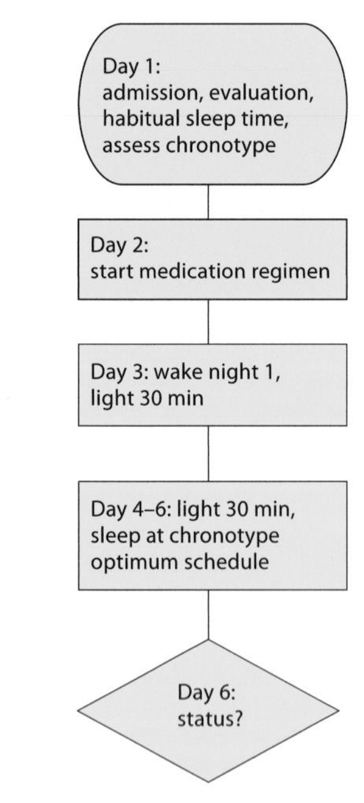

Flowchart 2

cording to MEQ-derived internal time is important in order to optimise phase stabilisation. Furthermore, morning light both stimulates alertness and potentiates the onset of the antidepressant effect.

4.6 Wake Therapy + Light Therapy + Sleep Phase Advance

We converge on the triple chronotherapeutic ensemble by adding a 3-day course of sleep phase advance therapy after one night of wake therapy and initiation of light therapy. Sleep phase advance therapy has been shown to sustain the acute improvement following a single night of sleep deprivation, thus forestalling relapse. As in the previous section, the procedure follows a similar course, illustrated in flowchart 3. After day 6, the procedure follows that of flowchart 1.

- Following wake therapy on day 3 and initiation of light therapy, the patient remains awake until a scheduled bedtime 5 h before habitual sleep onset. Sleep is allowed for the patient's habitual sleep duration (in the example, 8 h). If not already awake, the patient is awakened 4 h before the scheduled light therapy session on day 5.
- The goal is a minimum of 5 hours' sleep on sleep-phase-advance nights. If the patient awakens before the end of the scheduled sleep period and cannot resume sleep, he or she may rise and remain in low-level room light of approximately 30 lx at eye level (e.g. from a shaded reading lamp with an incandescent 25-watt bulb, and without overhead lights). An alternative is the use of blue-blockers under normal room light in the unit (fig. 19).
- From the time of scheduled wake-up to the time of the morning light therapy session, the patient remains in low room light of approximately 30 lx. The low level is required to forestall circadian rhythm phase delays during a procedure designed to foster phase advances.
- On day 5, bedtime is delayed by 2 h, placing it 3 h before habitual bedtime.
- On day 6, bedtime is again shifted 2 h later, placing it 1 h before habitual bedtime. This is the target for sleep onset under continued morning light therapy, since light therapy truncates habitual sleep and shifts the circadian clock earlier.
- As in the earlier procedures without sleep phase advance therapy, if there are only mild residual depressive symptoms on day 6, light exposure duration is increased from 30 to 45 min on day 7. If the patient remains depressed or there has been relapse after transient improvement, the chronotherapeutics protocol is further elaborated (examples below).

The recommended combination therapy protocol is illustrated in figure 24.

The protocol as described times the phase advance precisely, which may not always be possible.

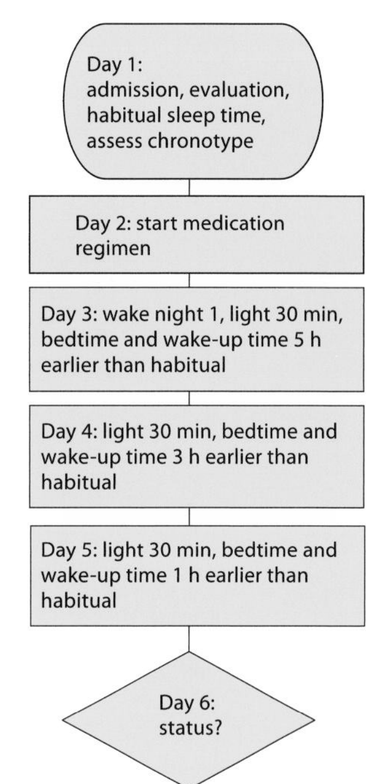

Flowchart 3

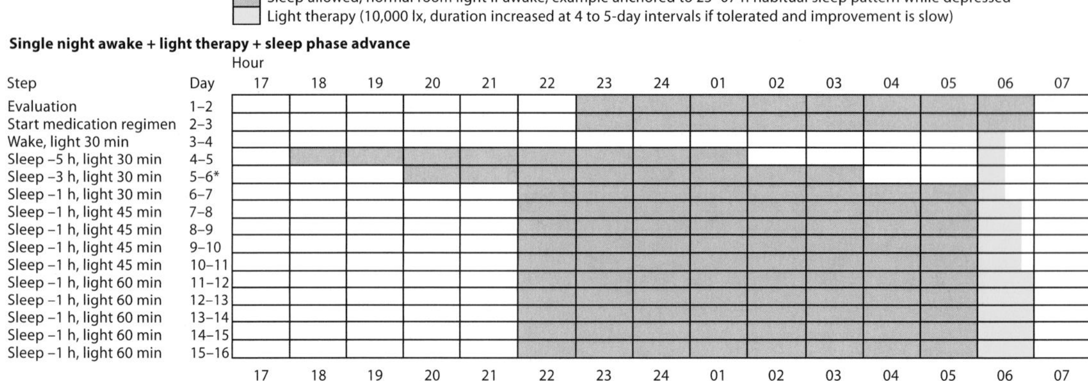

Fig. 24. Timeline for the same patient as in figure 22, encompassing spontaneous sleep while depressed, the starting time of morning light therapy from the MEQ algorithm, sleep deprivation, and a sleep phase advance. After earlier awakening on the nights of sleep phase advance, room light is kept low until the start of the light therapy session in order to forestall counteracting phase delay of the circadian clock.

Patients can also be left the freedom to choose when to go to bed (and be given a protected environment to enable early sleep), and be allowed to sleep as long as they like. This patient-friendly version of the protocol typically leads to a spontaneous phase advance of sleep onset by about 2 h (as measured by actimetry) [80]. However, in this flexible version of the phase advance protocol the patients are not required to wake up early, and in fact experience shows that they sleep longer in the recovery night after sleep deprivation. Clearly, however, in a research protocol, phase-advanced bedtime should be scheduled according to the patient's chronotype.

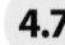

4.7 Three Alternate Nights of Wake Therapy + Light Therapy + Freely Chosen Sleep Phase Advance

The fully elaborated chronotherapeutics ensemble has been established in Milano as the procedure of choice for the treatment of by a major depressive episode without psychotic features in the course of bipolar disorder. It can also be used for patients who have been non-responsive at the earlier steps.

The complete triple wake protocol requires 6 days.

- Three nights of wake therapy alternate with 3 nights of freely chosen sleep phase advance.
- When wake therapy is repeated three times, we defer increasing light therapy duration from 30 min until day 9, giving precedence to the sleep-wake procedures, which are more likely to have an immediate effect.
- If the patient remains symptomatic, but with partial improvement at day 13, light therapy duration is increased to 60 min. Many patients with non-seasonal depression have settled on a 60-min maintenance regimen. In such long sessions, one may stand up and stretch for a few minutes, away from the light box, after half an hour of exposure.

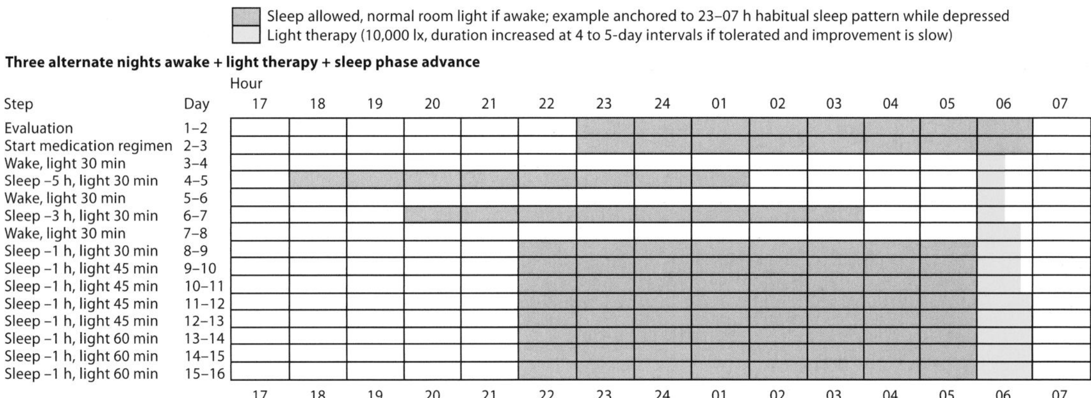

Fig. 25. Under the complete chronotherapeutics protocol, phase advanced sleep alternates with full nights awake, but moves back in 2-hour steps toward a maintenance sleep phase one hour earlier than at baseline.

4.8 Variations on the Theme

Not all hospitals are able or willing to set up the triple-wake-therapy protocol on their inpatient units, and will prefer to use a night awake either once, or once a week, or repeated only when a patient relapses or does not improve sufficiently. There are few published studies of such variations [82], and psychiatrists who use sleep deprivation are usually flexible in applying the procedure more than once to kindle response. Indeed, it was recognised early on that non-response to the first wake therapy can be followed by response on the second, and vice versa [20]. Cumulatively, there is increasing advantage up to three cycles, but two may be sufficient if remission is obtained and sustained by sleep phase advance therapy and light therapy.

A schematic proposed for full implementation of triple wake therapy, light and sleep phase advance is illustrated in figure 25.

In summary, the three main procedures can be combined flexibly as the clinician is able and the patient willing. Stabilising regular light therapy at the individual circadian optimum time is one pillar that should be maintained from the beginning. The second pillar is one or more nights of wake therapy, chosen according to patient needs and patient response. If possible, free choice of early bedtime is encouraged as a simple form of phase advance of sleep timing the night after sleep deprivation. Given the high level of sleepiness, this is usually no problem for the patients.

4.9 Maintenance Treatment

There are two separate issues: (a) to continue with light therapy at home, and (b) how to integrate further sleep deprivations, if indicated, and the feasibility of administering them on an outpatient patient basis (section 7).

If antidepressant treatment is discontinued during the expected duration of a depressive episode, it poses a distinct risk for relapse. Similarly, once discharged from acute hospital treatment, light therapy is conveniently continued at home on a maintenance basis and the advanced sleep schedule established should be maintained in the long term without a delay drift back to baseline. Ideally, patients should be provided with a light box to bridge the transition home, or the family given ordering information well before discharge, for purchase with timely delivery. The treating physician must receive a summary of the chronotherapeutics regimen used on the inpatient unit, so that compliance is maintained. See appendix 6 for an example of an information sheet to be handed out on discharge.

Attempts to discontinue treatment can result in rapid relapse, although resumption of treatment is effective within days. For non-seasonal cases, we recommend a full year of continuation treatment, following the general model for bipolar depression. This becomes a standard breakfast table routine (like qAM medication). For winter seasonal cases, discontinuation without tapering can be attempted starting in May, with resumption of light therapy for several more weeks if there is slumping or relapse. Continued clinician contact on an outpatient basis is a sine qua non.

4.10 Drug Tapering to Discontinuation

If patients have started a new antidepressant treatment in the last weeks and the results are not yet satisfactory, that treatment should never be stopped abruptly in favour of chronotherapeutics. Antidepressants take a lot of time (up to 2 months) to fully achieve their therapeutic potential, and the insufficient yet clinically relevant benefits during the first weeks are precious for the management of the case. Good clinical practice dictates tapering of drug discontinuation, since a sudden cessation of a not fully effective treatment during the first weeks can precipitate a clinical condition much worse than before: not only withdrawal effects, but also an acceleration of illness progression.

In case chronotherapeutics is initiated to speed up the recovery process, the psychiatrist should bear in mind that all antidepressant substances, with the exception of antidopaminergic drugs, are compatible with sleep deprivation, and thus can be continued during the chronotherapeutic treatment. If the psychiatrist wants to stop drugs anyway (for one of many possible reasons: unbearable side effects, etc.), it is strongly advisable to do it gently and to wait a couple of days before using wake therapy. This will avoid the potentially dangerous and unpredictable effect of adding the neurobiological correlates of drug withdrawal to the powerful neurobiological effects of wake therapy, as seen in Case Study 7.

Case Study 7
A Severe Error with Potentially Tragic Consequences

A 49-year-old female patient with bipolar 1 disorder was experiencing her fifth major depressive episode. Previous history showed one previous delusional episode treated with ECT because of severe psychotic and life-threatening symptoms, with good response to certain antidepressant drugs, but not to others. Long-term lithium salts treatment had appreciably reduced illness recurrence over her lifetime, but had not prevented the onset of the current episode four weeks previously. The psychiatrist who followed the patient in private practice started treatment with previously successful antidepressant drugs to which the patient had responded in previous episodes, and referred the patient for hospitalisation. The patient was admitted 10 days after beginning medication. Four days later, the clinical picture showed only negligible benefit: the antidepressants were discontinued, and the patient was administered a night of total sleep deprivation. During the night, the clinical picture worsened; the patient showed marked signs of psychic and somatic anxiety and became agitated. In the morning, with intense expressions of fear and anguish, she verbalised delusions of guilt and persecution, and suicidal thoughts. The acute situation was managed with intravenous benzodiazepines, and the patient eventually recovered after a typical 6-week course of antidepressant drug treatment. However, the wrong decision as to how to administer wake therapy elicited severe psychotic symptoms. In such cases, it is strongly advisable to continue the antidepressant drug and to initiate chronotherapeutics only after a careful assessment of the psychopathological picture that excludes any suspicion of ongoing psychotic symptoms. Beyond doubt, wake therapy works rapidly, but hurried psychiatrists can cause rapid worsening instead of rapid benefit [Benedetti].

A completely different scenario applies to patients who have been taking antidepressants for months without any clinical benefit, and want to try this new approach for their drug-resistant depression. Little or no benefit is expected from the old drugs, which are also likely to fail in sustaining the effects of sleep deprivation. In this case, mood stabilizers will be a better choice, particularly lithium salts, whose potential for treating resistant depression has been shown many times. These drugs can successfully overcome biological determinants of resistance to drug treatment. For example, lithium treatment successfully overcomes the negative bias against an antidepressant response due to unfavourable variants of the serotonin transporter promoter genotype [83].

The same principles apply to the tapering of drugs when a patient wants to replace them with light therapy. If the patient is experiencing poor or only moderate response to the antidepressant, light therapy should be added, with ascertainment of improvement before starting the drug taper. Although patients frequently request immediate drug discontinuation, they are unaware of the pitfalls of the withdrawal process.

5

Practical Details for Wake Therapy

5.1 Which Patients Are Suitable?

Wake therapy can be carried out in nearly all patients with a depression. A great deal of research – again, mostly in Europe – has shown that the response is found in all diagnostic subgroups [20]. Improvement has been seen in unipolar and even more dramatically in bipolar patients. In addition, mood in schizoaffective disorder and even negative symptoms in schizophrenia have been found to improve. Most of the clinical practice described here has been with bipolar patients, but we have sufficient experience with unipolar patients to affirm that the general principles are the same.

Exclusion Criteria

In an attempt to speed up response in a difficult-to-treat condition such as delusional depression, wake therapy alone has been administered to patients during a major depressive episode with psychotic symptoms. However, the patients experienced a worsening in delusions and their behavioural correlates, which indicates that wake therapy should be avoided in such cases. On the other hand, the melancholic non-delusional cognitive distortions typical of major depression are good prognostic indicators.

There is still little information about the effect of wake and light therapy in acutely suicidal patients. Discarded by all the trials dealing with the efficacy of antidepressants, these patients are usually treated with sedatives. Clinical experience, however, suggests that wake therapy is rapidly effective in suicidal cases, which of course requires close monitoring.

Going back to the early reports, Pflug [84] observed that in endogenous depression depressive mood improved more than psychomotor retardation, and argued that 'this is important in that it reduces the danger of suicide and allows us to treat outpatients with sleep deprivation'. Consistent with this observation, sustained improvements in the core cognitive distortions and mood congruent neuropsychological biases linked with depression have been reported after wake therapy, but further studies are needed to assess the effect of wake therapy in acutely suicidal patients.

Epilepsy should be regarded as a contraindication to wake therapy, given that (a) prolonged wakefulness is a known trigger for seizures, and (b) nothing is known about the interaction of antiepileptic medication and the therapeutic efficacy of wake therapy.

Finally, although generally well tolerated by healthy people, a night awake might be stressful for some. There are no specific contraindications to staying awake, but the procedure should be administered cautiously to people suffering from major medical illnesses (e.g. the depressed cancer patient).

5.2 Predictors of Response

Predictors of response to wake therapy include the same clinical and biological features that predict response to antidepressant drugs: presence of diurnal mood fluctuation, melancholic features, previous history of response to any treatments, etc. Bipolar patients have a higher response rate than unipolar patients. Some researchers consider the integrity of the dopaminergic system to be a prerequisite condition for response.

In the clinical setting, it will not be possible to measure functional brain correlates and predictors of antidepressant response. However, studies have consistently shown that the changes occurring with antidepressant response to wake therapy are closely similar to, but faster than, the changes observed under successful drug treatment (e.g. responders have higher baseline metabolism in the anterior cingulate cortex which decreases after treatment) [85, 86].

5.3 Medication Allowances and Contraindications

- Antidepressant medication should be continued as usual (most patients already come in on an SSRI).
- Bipolar patients on lithium should stay on lithium, while untreated patients should start lithium.
- There is little experience with other mood stabilisers (e.g. carbamazepine). The sedating effects of antiepileptics need to be evaluated.
- Antipsychotics and sedative drugs are counterindicated.
- Sleeping pills are not permitted on the night of wake therapy. Caffeine or modafinil may be used to promote wakefulness.

5.4 What to Tell Patients

As for all new treatments, patient education is crucial. The doctor describes the paradox that staying awake all night can be remarkably beneficial for treating depression, despite the usual wish of patients to have a pill to help sleep through the night. The paradox is explained by the biological nature of the illness. For example, early morning awakening in melancholia reflects an altered rhythmic state, yet the patient lacks the strength to get out of bed. When patients complete the chronotype questionnaire they realise that we are aiming to understand their personal sleep-wake rhythms and adjust treatment to their individual needs. If the patient remains dubious – 'Doctor, will I be able to stay awake all night? May I drink coffee?' – you reply 'Don't tell me you never stayed up a whole night! Of course, you may drink coffee if you need it'. One gets tired, but not as much as one would anticipate, and the improvement toward morning, coupled with light therapy, helps maintain wakefulness. Patients should be informed that they may feel worse again after the next night's sleep, but they will improve further following the next wake therapy. The various 'tricks' we apply – shifting the timing of sleep, using light therapy – are all aimed to prevent relapse.

5.5 Setting and Structure for the Night Awake

No special setting is required for wake therapy. In hospitals, the group living room can be used. Maintain normal daytime room light level. It might be useful at the beginning to check the room light intensities with a lux meter: approximately 300 lx at eye level is optimal. Availability of a warm meal and snacks during the night is important. If there is a garden, a good way of counteracting sleepiness is to have a short walk outside in the cool night air. Wake therapy can be carried out with a single patient; however, when there is more than one, the mutual 'adventure' eases the difficulties. Patients sometimes create a self-help group over the course of the night.

Patients who will undergo wake therapy should receive no sedative evening medication.

Activities are encouraged:

- Playing group games/cards
- TV, internet, DVD movies
- Cooking or eating a meal
- Talking and walking
- Stretching exercises (with video instructor)

To fight sleepiness:

- Patients should move around, and not remain seated for long periods
- Go for regular walks outside if possible
- Splash cold water on the face and hands to refresh
- Coffee, tea, caffeine candy and caffeinated soft drinks are allowed, ideally spread over the night in small portions; modafinil is an option (section 13.4.)
- The highest sleepiness is around 3–4 a.m., so be aware of possible naps and keep patients occupied

Mealtimes and quality:

- Allow patients to eat whenever hungry
- Serve one warm light meal during the night
- Allow multiple snacks as desired

5.6 Staff Monitoring

During the night awake, nursing staff closely monitors the patient with the aim of gently ensuring compliance and avoiding catnaps, reinforcing motivation and creating a warm human environment. It is important that the patients know they have ready access to staff in case of problems. The nurses should keep an eye open for anything that may go wrong, and engage the patient in conversation about changes in mood state that may occur during the night.

Monitoring the patients during wake therapy requires vigilance. Physicians and nurses are trained to observe, investigate and rate slowly occurring changes in the clinical picture, and become skilled in detecting the first signs of improvement. They need to catch any characteristics tending to deteriorate that could be a prelude to relapse. During wake therapy, they should anticipate changes over hours rather than weeks. On the way to overnight improvement, the patient will experience every possible transitional symptom between severe depression and euthymia, with the major therapeutic effect usually becoming apparent at dawn. Patients may also experience transient worsening over the course of the night. Mood fluctuations present a pretext to converse with the patients and reinforce adherence to the therapeutic protocol. The patients' perception of improvement will also reinforce the positive cognitive changes that are expected after successful treatment. The staff needs no special psychotherapeutic skills, but flexibility in engaging with patients is important.

We suggest that when implementing wake therapy procedures for the first time, an experienced psychiatrist stays awake together with the residents and nurses in order to provide an expert opinion on the rapidly unfolding psychopathological changes. For this first test of the method, it is advisable to select patients with good predictors of response. No specific instructions are required, because the psychopathological changes are the same as those seen during the course of remission, only more rapid. Teaching and learning will come with the observation of and interaction with the patient. Following standard procedure, the therapeutic staff will take all the usual precautions in case of unanticipated clinical changes (e.g. closer control if the patient begins to express suicidal thoughts).

5.7 Nurses on the Night Shift

The motivation of nurses or helpers on the night shift is a crucial element. They will need to have observed the successful response of several patients undergoing wake therapy to be convinced that it helps. Their enthusiasm is what supports the patients through the difficult dark hours after midnight, because the procedure is most challenging before the antidepressant effect begins to set in. However, if you put five people together with two nurses for a night awake, you do not need long training in psychotherapy – things will happen by themselves!

A hypomanic/manic switch is rare but possible: always have a physician on call.

5.8 Nurses on the Day Shift after Wake Therapy

Nurses manage the structure of the day after wake therapy as they managed the structure of the night. The treatment is not over at dawn. Wake therapy continues the entire day until early bedtime. Patients should not nap during the day. The same activities and exercise are as important here as during the night.

Thus, nurses are key figures to help patients respect changes in their biological rhythms that occur as a result of wake therapy and shield them from environmental interference as well. Their recovery sleep in the early evening needs to be protected from noise (e.g. talking outside rooms), since it occurs at a time when other patients on the unit are still engaged in daytime activities. Disruption of sleep by hospital routines (e.g. vital signs) should be avoided and delayed until the patient is awake.

5.9 Structure of the Day After

Hospital routine is usually rigid: to carry out successful chronotherapeutics, which involves sleep and wake at unusual times of day, the unit and personnel need to be more flexible and aware of problems.

During the day:

- Meal timing may need to be earlier than for the rest of the unit – the evening meal should be finished by 7 p.m.
- Napping is not allowed. Nurses should be aware that even the shortest nap could induce a sudden depressive relapse.
- In the afternoon, patients should avoid outdoor light and remain indoors until bedtime.

5.10 Phase Advance of Sleep following Wake Therapy

What time do we allow the patients to go to bed? The sleep phase advance is not difficult. It actually follows the natural inclination to go to bed early after being awake all night. The time of going to bed can be defined according to chronotype to tailor to individual differences, or be defined at 7:30 p.m. for all. Such a standardised phase advance of bedtime conforms to our individualised prescription for a patient who habitually sleeps at 12:30 a.m., i.e. a moderately late chronotype. Thus, for earlier chronotypes, it will not provide a full 5-hour phase advance (fig. 24).

In the formalised protocol with sleep phase advance, patients may not fall asleep spontaneously at the earlier bedtime on day 3, since the circadian clock will not have advanced by 5 h despite the accumulated sleep debt from the night before. Early evening low-dose melatonin would be a simple facilitator of the phase advance [87]. If sleep onset is difficult, it can be assisted with a short-acting benzodiazepine, e.g. triazolam 0.25 mg.

Depending on the patient's habitual sleep schedule and the season, the phase-advanced sleep may begin while it is still light outdoors or during dusk. Therefore, bedroom windows must be light-tight, using opaque curtains, shades or shutters.

In order to facilitate sleep when the unit is still active, the bedroom needs to remain quiet with the door closed (or cracked open for observation), and should not be shared. It is important to use a bedroom location as far as possible from group activities and the nursing station. Also, during recovery sleep after wake therapy and sleep phase advances, awakening a patient for vital signs must be avoided.

Thus, during the evening of a sleep phase advance:

- Clearly mark the patient's room as a 'silent area'.
- Check that there is no loud TV noise.
- Relatives and friends can visit only until 7 p.m., or earlier, if sleep onset is individualised per chronotype.
- Relatives and friends visiting other patients in the evening need to be informed of these 'quiet days' on the unit.
- Depending on timing in each hospital, nurses' shift changes may cause extra noise (e.g. 7 p.m., just when the patient is getting ready for bed).
- Bedtime at 7:30 p.m. or as individualised per chronotype (phase advance of sleep). Most patients in hospital experience a phase advance of their normal sleep-wake cycle anyway, just because hospital routine is earlier than at home.

Is the sleep phase advance necessary? It is a simple manipulation that has been shown to maintain the antidepressant response to wake therapy. Our strategy here is to combine all techniques we know to be complementary in order to potentiate clinical improvement. However, if the inpatient unit situation makes early bedtime impossible, the sleep phase advance can be eliminated from the chronotherapeutic ensemble.

5.11 The Doctor's Tasks

Before treatment begins, the physician explains to the patient all aspects of the treatment and gains assent. The chronotype questionnaire is filled out and the results are discussed in terms of disturbed rhythms.

Doctors usually do unit rounds in the morning and evening. With chronotherapeutics, they should go and look what is going on more often, since clinical state may change from hour to hour, particularly during the night of wake therapy.

Although it is not usual to administer rating scales to monitor clinical state in open treatment, daily ratings provide a useful benchmark for decision-making in the week-long chronotherapeutic progression. The abbreviated Hamilton 6-item scale of core symptoms has been useful in sleep deprivation studies, and requires but a moment of attention (appendix 4).

5.12 Is One-Time Wake Therapy Enough?

The number of nights required for wake therapy is still under discussion. Although the clinical improvement after a single night of wake therapy is remarkable, not all patients respond. This does not mean they will not respond to repeated nights of wakefulness. Some evidence suggests that repeated wake therapy has a kindling effect such that non-responders eventually switch. The best results have been achieved with the triple sleep deprivation protocol within 1 week.

Maintenance of the antidepressant response may be sufficient with light therapy and antidepressants. However, the possibility of administering a night of wake therapy during long-term maintenance is a treatment option.

5.13 Safety

Sleep deprivation has very few side effects. Remarkably, depressed patients do not get as tired as normal healthy subjects. Three alternate nights awake have been found safe in several studies. In bipolar patients, there have been occasional reports of switches into hypomania or mania. Patients with a prior history are monitored carefully and given prophylactic medication. Five percent of episodes of bipolar depression end with a manic switch when not under mood-stabilizing medication, and this rate increases to 10–15% with antidepressants. Current data on the effects of sleep deprivation in bipolar depression show an approximate 5% switch rate into mania and 6% into hypomania, which is no different from the rate found with serotonergic antidepressants. It should be noted that one third of switch patients who get a good night of recovery sleep (facilitated by benzodiazepines) will be immediately euthymic the next day and need no further treatment.

5.14 Special Conditions

- Drug-resistant patients: Response is expected to be lower (40–50% compared with 60–70% for drug responders), and relapse rate is higher. What differentiates these patients is that they do not maintain a benefit. Long-term follow-up has shown that a previous history of drug resistance negatively influences relapse rate. Nevertheless, these patients will experience some months of well-being (average 9 weeks), which is more than they would obtain under conventional drug treatment. Both physician and patient should not be surprised if and when relapse occurs. It is still unclear whether repeating the triple sleep deprivation procedure will lead to an extended period of euthymia. From a clinical point of view, there are no counterindications for repeating the protocol.
- Comorbid anxiety: Panic attacks will be expected to worsen during the night awake, but this will not reduce response. Susceptible patients need to be informed that they could experience a panic attack, but that nurses and doctors will be there to support them. Since such attacks rarely last longer than 10 minutes, we discourage intervention with benzodiazepines since that would promote sleepiness.
- Long-term neuroleptics: Patients on depot neuroleptics have a lower response to sleep deprivation. If possible, wait for washout to be complete and try again.

5.15 If There Is No Response

The rate of response to the combined chronotherapeutics protocol is high, but still there are non-responders. Since the trial requires only 1 week, the recourse is treatment-as-usual with antidepressant dose increments. Non-responders may still show improvement if the chronotherapeutics protocol is repeated after 1 week, in analogy to a series of ECT trials in treatment-resistant depression.

5.16 At the End of One Week of Chronotherapeutics

The combined chronotherapeutics protocol is designed to induce a fast and sustained antidepressant response in a high proportion of patients with major depression within 1 week. Thereafter, independent of whether they leave the hospital or remain longer, it is important to continue regular morning light therapy together with the antidepressant drug chosen for the individual patient.

After discharge, it is crucial that the responsible outpatient clinician be informed about the chronotherapeutic inpatient procedures that led to improvement, and the recommended maintenance regimen of light therapy. Patients should be given this information (see example in appendix 6) to discuss with their outpatient clinician. Moreover, both patients and physicians should be fully informed about the risk of relapse in order to schedule frequent assessments with rapid intervention in case of relapse. Should relapse occur within the first 3 months, it is important for the outpatient clinician to inform the attending hospital physician, so that long-term efficacy of the chronotherapeutic regimen can be evaluated.

5.17 In Conclusion

There is no difference in managing wake therapy and managing the illness itself. Patients with affective disorders are prone to relapse and recurrence, and the physician must always be prepared and prepare the patient for it. Whether relapse is rapid (the day after recovery sleep) or slow (days, weeks or months), the patient needs to understand the inherent periodicity of the illness. Good clinical practice means that the patient is reassured of clinical support in the long run.

6

Practical Details for Light Therapy

6.1 Criteria for Light Box Selection

This is an intricate section, since there are no official agencies regulating design with regard to safety and efficacy (the only requirements being electrical safety standards). Building and selling light boxes has grown into something of a cottage industry – nay, mass market – with many newer companies selling clinically untested apparatus, and several of the original companies introducing new models with unjustified claims for efficacy and ocular safety. There is a whole new set of concerns, and without federal or professional regulatory standards, the medical and scientific basis of the field is placed at risk by inadequate products and advertising.

We emphasise standards for light box design that consumers, doctors and insurance companies should keep in mind when selecting an apparatus to purchase. After careful consideration of three major factors – clinical efficacy, ocular and dermatologic safety, and visual comfort – we recommend the following criteria for light box selection:

- Any light box design should have been tested successfully in peer-reviewed clinical trials, or shown by independent laboratory measurements to match the field size, spectral content, intensity, UV screening and diffusion properties of well-tested units. (Unfortunately, manufacturers' specifications cannot always be trusted.)
- The light box should provide up to 10,000 lx of illumination at a comfortable sitting distance. Lux received at the eye falls off non-linearly and very rapidly with distance from the light box, thus the exact distance specified should be maintained. However, illuminance specifications by commercial parties are often missing or deceptive (based on measurements that do not subsume the whole visual field).
- The lamps should give off soft, broad-band white light rather than coloured light. There is no known therapeutic advantage so far established for 'full spectrum' lamps and blue (or bluish) lamps (section 6.4.), even though theoretical considerations – the blue wavelength-sensitive melanopsin-containing photoreceptors for the circadian system – make this a challenging prospect [88]. There appears to be a specificity for melatonin suppression, phase shifts, increased alertness and performance, and other ocular functions, although thus far not for antidepressant action. Interaction of melanopsin function with the classical photoreceptors responsive to longer wavelengths has been noted, but not fully elucidated. The premature marketing of blue augmentation in light therapy devices, with unproved claims for clinical efficacy, is a problem for the field. These devices cannot yet be recommended. At present, we recommend maintaining broad-spectrum white illumination, but filtering wavelengths lower than 450 nm to minimal levels in order to minimise risk of retinal damage.
- Fluorescent lamps should have a smooth diffusing screen that filters out ultraviolet (UV) radiation. Cumulative UV radiation, even at low levels, is harmful to the eyes and skin. The contour of the light bulbs should not be visually distinct.

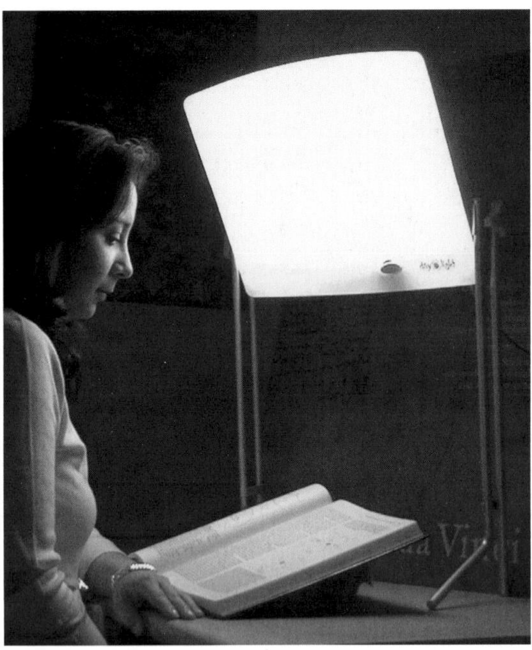

Fig. 26. A portable, lightweight light treatment apparatus that fulfils important safety and comfort criteria, and has been shown to be antidepressant in controlled clinical trials [89], e.g. Uplift Technologies, Model DL930 (Center for Environmental Therapeutics).

- The light should be projected downward toward the eyes at an angle to minimise aversive visual glare at high intensity.
- Field size matters: when using a compact light box, even small head movements may take the eyes out of the therapeutic range of light exposure.

The second generation of bright light boxes has a number of important improvements over early models: they are smaller, portable, with raised and downward-tilted placement of the radiating surface, a diffusion screen with nearly complete UV filtering, and high-output white fluorescent lamps with ballasts that eliminate flicker, yielding maximum illuminance of approximately 10,000 lx at a 30- to 33-cm distance. This configuration, with direction of gaze downward toward the table surface or toward a video monitor beneath the screen, provides non-glare illumination suitable for reading, and is generally well tolerated. Critical design features have not yet been specified or regulated, but miniature lighting devices, including lamps with blue augmentation, are not recommended.

6.2 Using the Light Box

Light therapy is a passive exercise. The patient sits facing the screen. Eye level looking forward is approximately two-thirds below the top of the screen, such that the preponderant illumination is from above. Screen height, table height and chair height should be adjusted accordingly. The treatment relies on peripheral retinal stimulation, which is fully achieved with a downward gaze. Eyes must remain open throughout the session. During the session, the distance of the head at 10,000 lx should be comfortably maintained; bending forward can produce excessive illumination, while moving back can lower the dose even below the therapeutic range. The patient engages in sedentary activities, including reading, writing, using a computer laptop, iPod, cell phone, eating breakfast, etc. With extended sessions (e.g. 60 min), the patient may stand up, stretch, use the bathroom, etc., returning to the session within a couple of minutes. If side effects of physical agitation or nausea emerge during a session, the light should be stopped immediately and the dosage lowered on subsequent days.

Likewise, the patient should time the session with a watch or clock in order to avoid overdose with excessive duration.

The treatment should be done under normal room light illumination, not in a dark room, in order to avoid aversive visual glare and headache.

6.3
Side Effects of Light Therapy

Adverse events are rare, and emergent sleep disturbances are usually related to the timing of light exposure and can be readily addressed. Side effects are minor and infrequent, and usually subside after a few days of treatment or with dose decreases (table 7).

6.4
Cautionary Notes about Bright Light Exposure

Light energy can interact with and damage skin and eye tissues, especially when a photosensitising molecule – whether from a drug or produced by the body – is bound within those tissues. The highest risk (for damage to the skin, and cornea and lens of the eyes) is from invisible, short-wavelength ultraviolet (UV) light, which has been filtered out of acceptable light therapy apparatus.

Long-term exposure to intense visible light in the blue range adjacent to the UV range may also pose a hazard to retinal photoreceptors and the pigment epithelium, which takes part in the photoreceptor renewal process. Above age 50, there is concern about blue-light exacerbation of age-related macular degeneration. Although some blue is an important component of white light exposure, lamps with relatively less blue (for example, soft-white fluorescents with colour temperatures in the range of 3,000–4,000 K) should be favoured over cool-white, daylight, or 'full spectrum' lamps (5,000 K and higher).

There are certain pre-existing medical conditions of eyes and skin that can also show photosensitisation reactions to intense visible light (table 8). In such cases, bright light therapy should be administered only under guidance and monitoring of an ophthalmologist or dermatologist, as indicated. Ophthalmologists should keep in mind that in some genetic retinal diseases the eyes become especially light sensitive.

Certain medications are known to photosensitise skin and/or retinal tissues. Examples in the visible range of light are summarised in table 9. Bright light therapy should not be used concurrently with these drugs. Melatonin may be used in conjunction with light therapy at opposite times of day (which is the correct way to use the two zeitgebers), but if used simultaneously, it can cause retinal photosensitisation.

Drugs that photosensitise primarily in the invisible UVA range (below the short-wavelength

Table 7. Infrequent side effects

- Mild visual complaints (eye irritability or fatigue)
- Nausea, dizziness
- Headache
- Insomnia after late evening light
- Premature awakening after morning light
- Hypomania in bipolar patients

Table 8. Pre-existing medical conditions of the eyes and skin that require caution

- Retinal dystrophies
- Age-related macular degeneration
- Porphyria
- Lupus erythematodes
- Chronic actinic dermatitis
- Solar urticaria

Table 9. Photosensitizing medications

- Psychiatric neuroleptic drugs (e.g. phenothiazine)
- Psoralen drugs
- Antiarrhythmic drugs (e.g. amiodarone)
- Antimalarial drugs
- Antirheumatic drugs
- Porphyrin drugs used in photodynamic treatment of skin diseases
- St. John's Wort (hypericum)

blue range) may also have a 'tail' of light absorption that extends into the lower visible blue light range, which could cause photosensitisation. Examples are tetracycline, diuretic drugs (e.g. hydrochlorothiazide), sulfonamide drugs and tricyclic antidepressants (e.g. imipramine, nortriptyline, desipramine, amitriptyline). If such a reaction is experienced or suspected, bright light therapy should be discontinued unless substitute medication is available, or it can be administered with protective measures under medical supervision.

6.5 Before Beginning Light Therapy

For normal healthy eyes, the exposure to bright white light is a physiological situation and does not inflict any overt damage to the skin, visual cells and pigment epithelium. Therefore, before beginning light therapy, pay attention to the following caveats:

- Medications that can enter the skin or retina and that absorb light in the visible range: These might cause photosensitisation with subsequent absorption of 'too many photons', leading to retinal damage. If a drug is in question, it is important to consult an ophthalmologist or dermatologist, as indicated.
- Certain inherited dystrophies of the retina that alter the visual pigments and can render the retina especially sensitive to visible light: If the patient suffers from an inherited retinal dystrophy and wants to use bright light therapy, consult an ophthalmologist.
- Age-related or other macular degenerations: For age-related macular degeneration (ARMD), genetic factors increase the risk of disease by about 50%. Patients with such risk factors, or those with several family members suffering from macular degeneration, should consult an ophthalmologist before using bright light therapy.
- Eyes of young patients up to an age of about 30–40 years transmit much more light to the retina than those of older patients: Thus, the eyes of younger patients are able to absorb generally higher light doses than those of older patients. Likewise, patients with lightly-pigmented irises (e.g. blue or green eyes) absorb higher proximal doses.
- Lenses in eyes of older patients become discoloured (yellowish) so that they filter more short-wavelength blue light than do the clear lenses in younger patients' eyes (and those with unfiltered lenses after cataract replacements): Indeed, blue-augmented light will have difficulty reaching the intended retinal target, making the use of such lamps questionable for older people. However, research into this issue is still ongoing.

6.6 In Conclusion

The practice of light therapy over the last 25 years, particularly in patients with primary affective disorders, but also for circadian rhythm sleep disorders, bulimia nervosa, Alzheimer's dementia, etc., has shown it to be a remarkably well-tolerated treatment modality with negligible side effects, given the caveats we have enumerated.

7

Outpatient Treatment Strategies

Given the importance of timing, regularity, and the unusual nature of the treatments – manipulating one's inner environment with wakefulness and one's external environment with light – hospitalisation for the full treatment ensemble is probably the most efficient method for seriously depressed patients.

However, given the favourable side-effect profile of these treatments, there is no counterindication to carrying them out at home. The main difficulty is adherence to the set protocols without continual guidance and monitoring by the clinician. In this section, we offer some guidelines for discussion with – and motivation of – the prospective outpatient.

7.1 Light Therapy

Light therapy is easier than sleep deprivation for outpatients. We have 25 years of experience giving patients light boxes to use as prescribed at home, with remarkable success in the majority of cases. Obviously, sitting in front of a light box involves more time and effort than taking a pill.

Methods to monitor compliance should be set up: the simplest is a log book to note the timing and duration of daily treatment sessions, sleep onset and offset, and daily mood and energy ratings (appendix 5). The record is then available for review at office visits, which provides a solid basis for dose and timing adjustments.

The importance of maintaining a consistent distance from the light box – an essential aspect of dosing – needs to be emphasised. The 'square root law' for reduced illuminance with distance teaches that even an extra 10 cm distance through displacement of a chair or table can reduce the dose received by half (instead of 10,000 only 5,000 lx, for example). In the outpatient setting, 30 min can usually be fitted into the morning schedule; 60 min is more difficult and requires careful planning (if necessary, together with the family so that they realise the importance of regular sessions).

The importance of timing to maximise the therapeutic effect also needs to be emphasised. This is often problematic with delayed and long sleepers, who find it particularly difficult to get up for light treatment scheduled somewhat before their habitual wake-up time. One way of dealing with this is to begin the light therapy at the usual time of getting up, and then start it 15 min earlier every few days. Morning light advances the biological clock, so that this gradual shift will make it easier to get up as the sessions continue, until the targeted treatment time is reached. If wake-up time and light therapy are moved earlier too quickly, there can be a sudden relapse into the delayed pattern. Indeed, the patient may start to go back to sleep after the treatment session.

Light therapy has been widely used as monotherapy in outpatients (in particular, for SAD), but is more commonly combined with standard antidepressant medication in non-seasonal depression. The severity of seasonal variation is conveniently evaluated using the Personal Inventory for Depression and SAD (PIDS-SA, appendix 2; PIDS, appendix 7). If a response to light does not emerge within 4 days, the duration of exposure is gradually increased up to 60 min. If the response to light is strong, there is a prospect for reduced reliance on drugs, even longstanding ones. In the words of a psychopharmacologist colleague, 'No one wants to take drugs'. That goal can be a powerful motivator for many outpatients.

Finally, the same screening procedures used for inpatients (e.g. ocular disease, photosensitising medication) should be a part of outpatient management (appendix 7). If the patient has not had a routine eye examination in more than 2 years, it is wise to require one in order to rule out pre-existing ocular pathology that might otherwise be attributed to light treatment.

7.2 Wake Therapy

Sleep deprivation is more difficult to execute at home, but has succeeded individually and in studies. Ideally, a partner or friend should stay up with the patient all night to help sustain wakefulness and pass the slow hours after midnight. This person should keep careful watch that no naps occur. One patient in Greece regularly went dancing every Saturday night with her husband; she remained euthymic. One psychoanalyst in New York was able to stay awake reading on Saturday nights and did not slump till Thursday. A manager in Italy treated her recurrent depression with the full triple-wake protocol, and could successfully combine repeated wake therapy nights with morning work commitments.

An ideal solution, not yet implemented, would be to institutionalise outpatient wake therapy by having a room (in a private practice, for example) where patients come to stay up all night. The wake therapy would be scheduled on specific days of the week, so that several patients are present as a group and can profit from mutual interaction through the night. A night nurse would be present to guide and support the patients. The office should be near public transport, to accommodate easy arrival and morning departure without the need to drive. (Driving immediately after a night awake is counterindicated.) The room should be large enough, with a kitchen for cooking meals and having snacks, a bathroom, and the opportunity to go outside for an invigorating walk. Such a dedicated facility for outpatient wake therapy would take the monitoring burden off family members and help to organise proper scheduling of the chronotherapeutic regimen.

As with the combined therapeutic procedures for inpatients, the rapid response to wake therapy can be stabilised with light therapy at the end of the night of sleep deprivation.

8 Range of Chronotherapeutic Indications

We have focused on chronotherapeutics for the treatment of major depression. Sleep deprivation has an antidepressant effect in many forms of affective disorders, independent of age and aetiology, and improves the negative symptoms in schizophrenia [20]. In this sense, it is specific for treating the spectrum of depressed mood and cognition. In contrast, light therapy is applicable in a wide variety of psychiatric disorders, not just depression, as summarised in section 1.8. [27, 32, 90]. We need to emphasise that light therapy goes beyond SAD and is particularly recommended for non-seasonal depression. It is encouraging that light therapy is effective even for chronic depression of more than 2 years' duration and in therapy-resistant patients whose only conventional alternative may be ECT.

We know now that circadian rhythm sleep disturbances in other psychiatric illnesses may also be treated with light therapy, melatonin, or both, as adjuvants to drugs. Even though we do not know much about the causal links in the circadian rhythm sleep disturbances/psychiatry axis, it may well go in both directions (table 10). Poor sleep-wake cycle entrainment could lead to psychopathology in vulnerable individuals. Thus, stronger circadian entrainment may improve clinical symptoms, independent of aetiology.

A neural system governed by the master clock in the SCN, with multiple peripheral clocks (fig. 3), offers unlimited opportunity for internal and external desynchronisation. The therapeutic process requires that the SCN synchronise to the environmental day-night cycle, that oscillators in peripheral organs (liver, gut, adrenal) must follow suit, and that the panoply of peripheral oscillators achieve mutual synchrony. Achieving a steady stable state can be a slow process, requiring sustained, regular 24-hour synchronising zeitgeber input (light, dark, mealtimes, exercise, social contact, medication) [44]. Beyond the regularity of individual daily zeitgebers, their timing needs to be coordinated to support resynchronisation.

The domain of tested chronotherapeutic applications is still nascent, but already wide.

Table 10. The circadian-sleep/psychopathology axis

- Most psychiatric illnesses are accompanied by sleep disturbance
- Some disorders have sleep disturbance as a diagnostic criterion (e.g. major depressive disorder)
- Sleep disturbance may precede the illness episode (e.g. a spontaneous night awake at the switch into mania)
- Circadian sleep-wake cycle disorders have high psychiatric comorbidity

8.1 Antepartum Depression

Both open-label [91] and controlled studies [35] have successfully employed light therapy for major depression during pregnancy, which offers a safe somatic treatment alternative to antidepressant drugs regardless of whether the woman has a history of seasonal depression. Both efficacy and side effects have been shown to be dose-dependent [35]. For example, a non-responder to 60 min of 7,000 lx light administered upon awakening for 5 weeks showed full remission when session duration was increased to 75 min. A responder who developed irritable hypomania under the same initial treatment conditions became depressed when duration was reduced to 45 min, but responded without hypomania when duration was increased to 50 min. Although larger-scale trials are needed, morning light therapy is a viable option for treatment of antepartum depression.

Some patients who have responded to antepartum light therapy have bridged it to the postpartum period, with good subjective effect, although clinical trials are still pending.

Preliminary data suggest that partial sleep deprivation can alleviate antepartum depression and be well tolerated by the patients [92].

8.2 Premenstrual Dysphoric Disorder

Patients with both seasonal and non-seasonal premenstrual dysphoric disorder (PMDD) or milder premenstrual syndrome (PMS) have responded favourably to 1 week of light therapy during the luteal phase [93]. However, timing and dose were non-specific. By contrast, a 2-month study using 10,000 lx, 30-min evening light during the luteal phase found significant improvement relative to a dim light control, with alleviation of both depressed mood and physical symptoms [94].

The recommendation of evening light therapy for PMDD stands counter to the morning light protocol usually indicated for affective disorders. Adequate trials are lacking to test the specificity of this recommendation, which was originally based on the assumption that circadian rhythms advance in the luteal phase and require resetting to a later hour. Clinically, a PMDD patient who oversleeps, or has difficulty waking up, might best begin with morning light therapy. We consider the chronotherapeutic approach especially valuable for women who have not responded to medication.

Partial sleep deprivation, both in the early and late part of the night, has been shown to successfully ameliorate mood in patients affected by premenstrual dysphoria. As in the case of light therapy, however, the pattern of response did not follow usual observations in other types of depression, and best improvements were seen after recovery sleep rather than after the night of restricted sleep [95].

8.3 Bulimia Nervosa

Many patients with bulimia nervosa manifest seasonal exacerbation of symptoms. An open treatment study yielded average reductions of 46% in binge eating and 36% in purging, along with 56% reduction in depression scale scores [96]. A controlled study showed marked superiority of morning bright light therapy (30 min, 10,000 lx) over dim light, for both mood and bulimic symptoms [97]. Even in bulimic patients without winter depression, morning bright light therapy diminished bingeing and purging more than under a dim light placebo [97]. The data thus augur well for the use of light therapy in bulimia with or without concomitant winter depression.

8.4 Attention Deficit/Hyperactivity Disorder

There is a high incidence of winter depression with hypersomnia, indicative of circadian rhythm phase delay, in patients with ADHD [98, 99]. A 3-week open trial of morning light therapy (10,000 lx, 30 min) in ADHD with or without seasonal mood pattern produced clinically significant improvement in core ADHD symptoms and neuropsychological deficits [100]. Improvement was unrelated to depression status, with greatest benefit in patients who showed increased morningness on the MEQ, a proxy measure of circadian rhythm phase advance [100].

8.5 Dementia

Although many attempts with light therapy in these difficult patients have produced mixed results, recent work shows great promise. One 3-week trial has compared morning, evening, and daylong enhanced room light exposure [101]. Both morning and all-day exposure advanced the circadian sleep-wake cycle with increased sleep duration. As expected, evening light delayed the sleep cycle without sleep improvement. The orderliness of results – which was most evident in the most severely demented subgroup – warrants further development of circadian lighting regimens in long-term care facilities.

A larger study followed patients for more than 3 years on an all-day lighting regimen administered alone or supplemented with melatonin, melatonin administered alone, or treatment-as-usual [40]. Increased lighting enhanced the stability and amplitude of the rest-activity rhythm, improved mood and reduced cognitive deterioration. The best results were obtained with light combined with melatonin; melatonin monotherapy, at least in the supraphysiological dose used here, resulted in mood deterioration.

A 3-week trial of dusk-to-dawn simulation in demented elderly patients, administered at bedside and time-anchored individually to each patient's sleep-wake cycle, advanced nocturnal sleep onset by more than 1 h, with commensurate increases in sleep duration and nocturnal quiescence [39].

8.6 Parkinson's Disease

Though it might be hypothesised that light therapy would reduce the depressive symptoms often seen in Parkinson's disease, it would be surprising also to obtain improvement in core motor symptoms, which is the aim of dopamine replacement therapy. A 2-week pilot trial of 12 patients who received presleep light therapy produced clinically significant reduction in bradykinesia and rigidity – but not tremor – in parallel with an antidepressant effect [102]. Patients could not tolerate illuminance levels above 1,500 lx, and the choice of evening light was based on the presumption of advanced melatonin onset and peak phases, which are especially prominent under dopamine replacement therapy. Despite such phase advances, sleep onset insomnia is prevalent in these patients, yet evening light paradoxically served to reduce sleep onset latency. The relative advantage of morning light therapy awaits testing. Of note, under light therapy many patients were able to sustain up to 50% dose reduction of dopaminergic medication without loss of symptom control, which offers promise for alleviating treatment-emergent levadopa-related motor complications.

The potential usefulness of wake therapy in Parkinson's disease is controversial. Patients often experience a rapid amelioration of mood and motor symptoms during a night awake, but a 'sleep benefit' due to replenishing presynaptic dopamine stores and a wake-induced symptomatological worsening due to a depletion of brain dopamine have also been described. Caution is recommended in using this treatment [103].

8.7 Shift Work and Jet Lag Disturbance

Disruption of the circadian timing system is ubiquitous in rotating and nightshift work and after long distance jet travel across time zones. The trigger is external and the symptoms are not indicative of endogenous pathology, in contrast with the disorders and illnesses that are our focus here. Endogenous factors may certainly play a role in susceptible individuals. The rapid time zone transition eastward can trigger a manic switch, westward a depressive episode. A patient with 35 years of recurrent winter depression returned to the US after 6 months in Australia (switching seasons and time zones), and entered into a prolonged non-seasonal depression. Even without a lifetime history of affective disorder, transmeridian flight can disrupt mood and cognitive function in addition to the common jet-lag symptoms of digestive disruption, sleep difficulties and waves of daytime fatigue.

Jet lag is transient, though the symptoms are uncomfortable and may last several days or even weeks [104]. Appropriate light exposure (either from lamps or outdoors) and light avoidance (with blue-blocking eyeglasses) can be calculated from the phase shifts required to resynchronise: the timing depends on the direction and number of time zones crossed. Often, melatonin is used, particularly for the more difficult phase advance; its soporific properties also help in sleeping during the flight.

Shift work studies – primarily laboratory simulations – have focused on minimising the magnitude and duration of symptoms upon entering the shifts [104], or arranging appropriate phase adjustments in preparation for the shifts using combinations of timed melatonin, light treatment, dark exposure, blue-blocking eyeglasses, and sleep scheduling [105]. Given the complexity of shift work schedules and countervailing social demands of the real world, there are many obstacles for implementing such a program by industry. This is a major challenge for applied chronobiology. Short of active interventions, one practical approach takes into account the individual worker's chronotype: late chronotypes adapt better to evening and night shifts, early chronotypes to the morning shift.

9

Light Therapy for Children and Adolescents

Light therapy can be used to treat mood and sleep disorders throughout the entire life span. The indications remain the same as for prescribing antidepressants. What should be specifically addressed when treating childhood and adolescent depression?

The prevalence of SAD is correlated with age/puberty, is higher in postpubertal girls, and in adolescents is of the same order as in adults (around 2%) [106]. Children usually present symptoms more on the energy dimension (fatigue, difficulties getting up in the morning, school problems, lack of sociability, irritability) rather than low mood in the winter months. Thus, parents and doctors should be aware that seasonal problems are manifested in sleep difficulties and low energy and school performance rather than by obvious depression, and consider light as an aid to improve them. Paediatric SAD has been successfully treated with light in controlled studies [107] and in everyday practice. Few side effects have been reported. The main problem has been compliance (regular daily light exposure, including Sundays, is required). Sitting at a light box for 30 min is particularly onerous for children under 6 years, and regular outdoor morning activities should be considered instead if the sun has risen by that hour.

Adolescence is also the time when the biological clock shifts forward. Teenagers delay their bedtimes and would like to delay their wake-up times as well [108]. The extreme condition known in sleep medicine as delayed sleep phase disorder (DSPD) can be somewhat held in check by morning light given to advance circadian sleep propensity [109]. This syndrome is not easy to treat, since adolescents cannot easily get up early for their light exposure, and any irregularity (leaving out morning light for a few days) leads to return of the delayed sleep phase. Strategically, they can begin the light therapy at their normal wake-up time, and then shift it 15 min earlier every few days. The advancing effect of light on the biological clock encourages earlier bedtime, thus easing the treatment regimen.

Adolescents often resist attempts to resynchronise bedtime because of the peer pressure to socialise late into the night, whether in person or online. Despite his depression, and loss of class time due to DSPD, a 17-year-old objected, 'Earlier sleep is for 40-year-olds, not for us!' Additionally, many are embarrassed that they need treatment, do not talk about it, and even hide their light boxes from their friends.

There is current major concern by faculty, administration and health service units about an increase in college students' psychiatric and sleep disturbances. Mary Susan Esther, President of the American Academy of Sleep Medicine, senses a core problem of delayed sleep phase: 'Having walked on these campuses, I can tell you it's changed a lot. It used to be fairly quiet by 2 a.m. Now that is sort of midday. That's the part I worry about most' (New York Times, January 15, 2009).

Many children and adolescents with attention deficit/hyperactivity disorder (ADHD) have a primary sleep disorder with delayed circadian phase. DSPD in childhood is often mistakenly diagnosed as psychological insomnia or attributed to inappropriate behaviours. Parents and doctors need to recognise altered biological clock function as a primary factor underlying late sleep times. Such awareness might increase the appropriate treatment – either morning light or evening melatonin treatment, or both. Many of the symptoms reflect what chronobiologists call 'social jet lag' – an internal desynchronisation between required bedtime and the time point when the individual is actually biologically ready for sleep [110].

Norman Rosenthal described a case with a triple diathesis: winter depression, DSPD and ADHD in a teenage girl [111]. The three comorbid disorders, which have their source in circadian rhythm phase delay, were successfully treated by light therapy.

While light therapy improves depressive symptoms in bulimia nervosa (seasonal or nonseasonal), it also reduces binge and purge frequency in adults. Bulimic adolescents are now also beginning to use the treatment.

Compliance with 30 min of morning light therapy before school can be an extreme challenge for children and adolescents who are already late getting up for school. Automated dawn simulation in the bedroom in the final period of sleep may offer an effortless timesaving solution.

Melatonin has been used successfully as an evening zeitgeber in the evening to treat delayed, free-running, and irregular sleep-wake cycle disorders in developmentally disabled children with cognitive and visual impairment [109, 112]. It may be useful also for a wide variety of delayed sleep manifestations in children, regardless of psychopathology. However, given the possible interaction of exogenous melatonin with development of the reproductive axis (endogenous levels plummet after puberty), chronic melatonin treatment may be counterindicated.

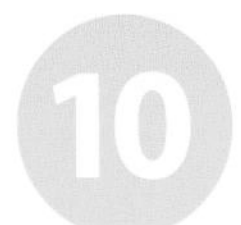

Light and Wake Therapy for Older Patients

Light therapy has potential widespread utility in older individuals. Although SAD prevalence declines with age after 50, the disorder can persist throughout life, and light therapy remains an effective intervention. Light therapy for non-seasonal geriatric depression has mixed reviews, although a trial is indicated if there is a sleep-wake cycle disturbance. Regardless of depression, many older individuals develop advanced sleep phase disorder (ASPD) with sleep onset in the evening and awakening with full alertness hours before dawn. They often report the strangeness of being wide awake as the world sleeps, and worse, of having nothing to do in this dark part of the night (*l'heure du loup* – the hour of the wolf).

Ageing affects the circadian system and sleep. Changes occur at the level of photic input to the retina and in the SCN itself. The eye can undergo a variety of degenerative processes, some of which diminish the amount and the spectral composition of light input, and thus the retinal signal to the SCN. After age 40, transmission declines as the ocular media become cloudy, a natural and normal ageing process. In later years, lens protein undergoes structural changes leading to a yellowish hue that attenuates short wavelength input. Cataract formation provides an additional filter, and macular degeneration degrades transduction of the residual input.

The ageing SCN shows reduced neuronal activity and manifests itself in a diminished amplitude of circadian efferents to all downstream functions, including melatonin production and the sleep-wake cycle [113, 114]. This degeneration is most obvious in Alzheimer's disease (AD) [113]. Swaab et al. [113] prescribed the rule for activating the remaining function of the SCN – *Use It or Lose It!* It is equally applicable to normal ageing to enhance SCN function by whatever means possible, prominently by enhanced zeitgeber input [114]. Correct timing and sufficient exposure to light are general objectives for healthy ageing.

Behavioural factors also influence the older person's light exposure. Many live under extremely dim room lighting, and are less likely than younger people to go outdoors during the day. In particular, dim evening room light promotes circadian rhythm phase advances and early sleep onset.

If the older depressed patient has a normal or delayed sleep-wake cycle, the rules of morning light exposure according to the MEQ chronotype apply. However, for those with abnormally early sleep onset, early morning awakening, or both, evening light exposure in the hour before sleep can serve to normalise sleep onset, often with mood improvement. Even when effective in early clinical trials, most elderly subjects decided against continuation treatment; they found light therapy uncomfortable/glaring, and the regimen distracting from habitual evening activities. With improvements of light diffusion and angled presentation from above the line of sight, and enhancement of dose to 10,000 lx for reduced session duration, newer apparatus may make this treatment option more acceptable.

In older patients with insomnia, increased daytime light exposure served to increase nocturnal melatonin secretion, with improvement of sleep initiation and consolidation [115]. A combination of all-day enhanced lighting with evening melatonin administration halted cognitive decline in AD, and improved sleep continuity and mood [40]. This protocol increased intensity of overhead lighting in the group room where most of the patients spent their day, since previous trials had difficulty keeping these patients in front of a light box. Another option that relieves the patient – and nursing staff – of behavioural involvement with the treatment regimen is automated dusk-to-dawn simulation in the bedroom. A 3-week pilot study achieved a phase advance of sleep greater than 1 h accompanied by longer sleep duration and reduced restlessness [39].

Apart from light exposure, evening melatonin administration can benefit sleep timing and quality in ageing individuals. If the sleep cycle is delayed, early evening melatonin can serve to advance and stabilise phase. If the sleep cycle is advanced, however, melatonin should be given only shortly before the desired sleep time, in which case the positive effects are due to the direct, sleep-inducing properties of melatonin and not its phase-shifting properties (section 12.1.).

As for wake therapy, there were 'better-than-anticipated' antidepressant effects in elderly patients in the earliest work [116], which have been repeatedly confirmed. Increasing age does not hamper response to wake therapy, and the indications and practical considerations are the same as for younger patients.

By contrast, patients with dementia have shown no benefits from wake therapy. Indeed, a single night awake has been proposed as a tool for differential diagnosis between late life depression and dementia. However, clinical experience suggests a difference between the positive and negative predictive power of this probe: although an abrupt increase in mood can well confirm the diagnosis of geriatric depression, a lack of response is uninformative.

The Visually Impaired: More Sleep Disturbances, More Depression

Psychiatrists are usually not in close contact with ophthalmologists, and vice versa. However, we need an active dialogue. We know there is a circadian clock in the eye as well as the SCN (fig. 3), actively gating the photic signal. Light is now recognised not only as crucial for vision, but as the major zeitgeber for circadian rhythms and sleep. Thus, it follows that that there are different degrees of circadian rhythm sleep disorder and possibly mood disturbances along the spectrum of visual impairment. Still to be established is whether loss of sensory visual perception includes loss of function of the melanopsin-containing ganglion cells, beyond peripheral reduction of the light input signal.

Circadian rhythm sleep disorders are manifested in three forms of visual deficit: (a) absolute, without any photoreception and signal transmission following ocular enucleation; (b) perceptual blindness, where a subset of patients maintain circadian light sensitivity and melatonin suppression by light; and (c) progressively reduced light perception or partial blindness, as may occur during cataract formation, glaucoma, diabetic retinopathy and macular degeneration. The resulting sleep disorders are either free-running – in which the circadian clock is no longer entrained to the 24-hour day – or abnormally entrained, usually very late (DSPD), but occasionally very early (ASPD).

Patients with progressive visual loss are more vulnerable to sleep disturbance than those with normal ocular transduction [43, 117]. Sleep-wake timing disorders occur in 50% [118] to 70% [Remé, unpubl. data] of blind patients. Abnormal melatonin rhythms are more common in patients who lack conscious light perception (no light perception, NLP) than in those with residual light perception (light perception, LP) [43, 119]. In a French survey, 83% of respondents reported at least one sleep problem; free-running sleep disorder occurred in 17% of NLP compared to 8% in sighted controls [120]. A New Zealand study found that blind and visually impaired patients experienced more sleep disorders and daytime somnolence than sighted controls [121]. The highest incidence of sleep timing problems occurred in the NLP group: 26% drifting sleep patterns versus 4% in sighted controls. Likewise, a Swiss survey found the greatest sleep disturbance in those with binocular visual acuity loss greater than 90%, followed by those with 40–90% binocular acuity loss. Taken together, sleep disturbance was nearly five times more frequent given such loss in visual acuity than in controls [Remé, unpubl. data].

Bilaterally enucleated patients are nearly all free running [43, 119]. In many cases, irregular sleep is so ingrained that it is not perceived as something to complain about. In some cases, lack of a structured daily schedule may result in compensatory napping and erratic bedtimes. Sleep disturbance might arise from factors secondary to blindness, such as unemployment and unstructured daily routines (reduced social synchronisers). Some NLP patients may entrain through residual photoreception by melanopsin-containing ganglion cells. Thus, enucleation should be avoided whenever possible in order to maintain non-visual light detection.

Glaucoma leads to a partial reduction of melanopsin-containing ganglion cells, which may affect both circadian and extra-circadian (e.g. pupillary reflex) non-sensory visual functions [122]. Patients with glaucoma have lower plasma melatonin levels, decreased light sensitivity (reduced melatonin suppression after light exposure) and higher variability in the DLMO [123]. Similar findings can be expected for cataract patients – a different pathology reduces the amount of light reaching the retina, and hence the photic signal to the SCN. (In contemporary medical practice, lens replacement usually takes place before advanced stages of cataract formation, so the numbers affected are now relatively small.)

Sleep disturbance is of course associated with mood disorders, though cause and effect are not clear. One study found depression more prevalent with increasing glaucoma severity [124]. More than 25% of patients with age-related macular degeneration met the DSM-IV criteria for depressive disorder, and had significantly greater levels of general and vision-specific disability than non-depressed ARMD patients [125]. Depressed patients with retinitis pigmentosa had poorer vision-related functions than RP patients without depression, which could not be explained by reduced visual acuity [126]. Cataract surgery significantly improved vision-related quality of life, cognitive function and depressed mood in elderly patients [127].

Deficits in light input to the retina, or the retinal response to light, should not be taken to imply that the therapeutic solution is necessarily intense stimulation with light, which is often counterindicated in degenerative retinal disease. Properly structured schedules of dim illumination – as in dusk-to-dawn simulation (section 2.3.) – can maintain entrainment, elicit phase shifts and melatonin suppression, and positively influence mood, sleep timing and quality. Such protocols have never been tried as a treatment for the sleep and mood problems of visually impaired patients with residual circadian light perception.

Research has focused on use of exogenous melatonin as zeitgeber, which does not depend on circadian photoreception. Patients with or without conscious light perception or residual melanopsin function can respond to timed melatonin treatment with entrainment of the biological clock to the 24-hour day and improved sleep quality, sleep timing and quality of life [43, 128]. Thus, psychiatrists should be aware that visually impaired or blind patients presenting with depression and/or sleep disturbances are likely to suffer from a circadian rhythm problem, and can be offered melatonin treatment (section 12), though the specifics of dosage, formulation (controlled release vs. bolus) and individual timing are still under investigation.

Endogenous and Exogenous Melatonin

Melatonin, the hormone secreted by the pineal gland, has been the subject of exaggerated, unsubstantiated claims during recent years. A veritable melatonin mania in the media and injudicious advertising has clouded the actual extraordinary role(s) this hormone is known to play. On the one hand, there is an entire area of research related to its antioxidant, free-radical-scavenging properties (in particular, in terms of anti-ageing). On the other hand, our Manual focuses on its role in transducing the solar day into a hormonal signal of 'biological night' [9, 10]. The 24-hour melatonin cycle informs the brain and body of nighttime, and also the time of year, by transducing night length into the duration of nightly secretion [9].

Melatonin peaks when core body temperature, alertness, and cognitive performance are at their lowest [129] (fig. 27). The endogenous melatonin rhythm is closely associated with the circadian component of the sleep propensity rhythm (process C, section 1.4.). In a 32-hour laboratory study of sustained wakefulness, the time course of neurobehavioural performance is characterised by fairly stable levels throughout the first 16 h, followed by deterioration during the phase of melatonin secretion. As illustrated on the left hand side of figure 27, the evening rise in melatonin triggers changes in objective markers of sleepiness, namely a slowing of eyeblink rate, increase in slow eye movements, and epochs of stage 1 sleep occurring despite the injunction to stay awake. The dynamics of slow eye movements and EEG activity are phase locked to changes in neurobehavioural performance (fig. 27, right) and lag the plasma melatonin rhythm. Increased subjective sleepiness is associated with a rise in the number of performance lapses and a decline in cognitive throughput and memory recall. It becomes clear that any circadian misalignment can trigger a shift in sleepiness and performance.

If sleep occurs outside the biological night, its quality and duration are compromised. That is why endogenous melatonin is understood as a hormone which facilitates and reinforces sleep and other nighttime physiologic functions. An example from a 'forced desynchrony' protocol (fig. 28), where subjects went to sleep at every circadian phase over a period of weeks, shows that sleep continuity is extremely high (with minimal wakefulness in sleep episodes) during the period of melatonin secretion, and declines during the biological day, when melatonin is absent [130].

12.1 The Physiological Effects of Melatonin

Light plays a dual role: first, as a zeitgeber for the biological clock, i.e. as a synchronising and phase-shifting agent, and second, it has acute (direct) physiological effects that increase alertness.

Melatonin also plays a dual role. First, it has established zeitgeber properties, with phase advances in the afternoon and evening before endogenous melatonin onset, and phase delays in the second half of the night through the morning [10, 15]. This phase response curve (fig. 6) is roughly opposite to that of light, which induces delays in the evening after melatonin onset and advances in the latter hours of sleep and early morning. Secondly, exogenous melatonin has acute (direct) effects that increase sleepiness and

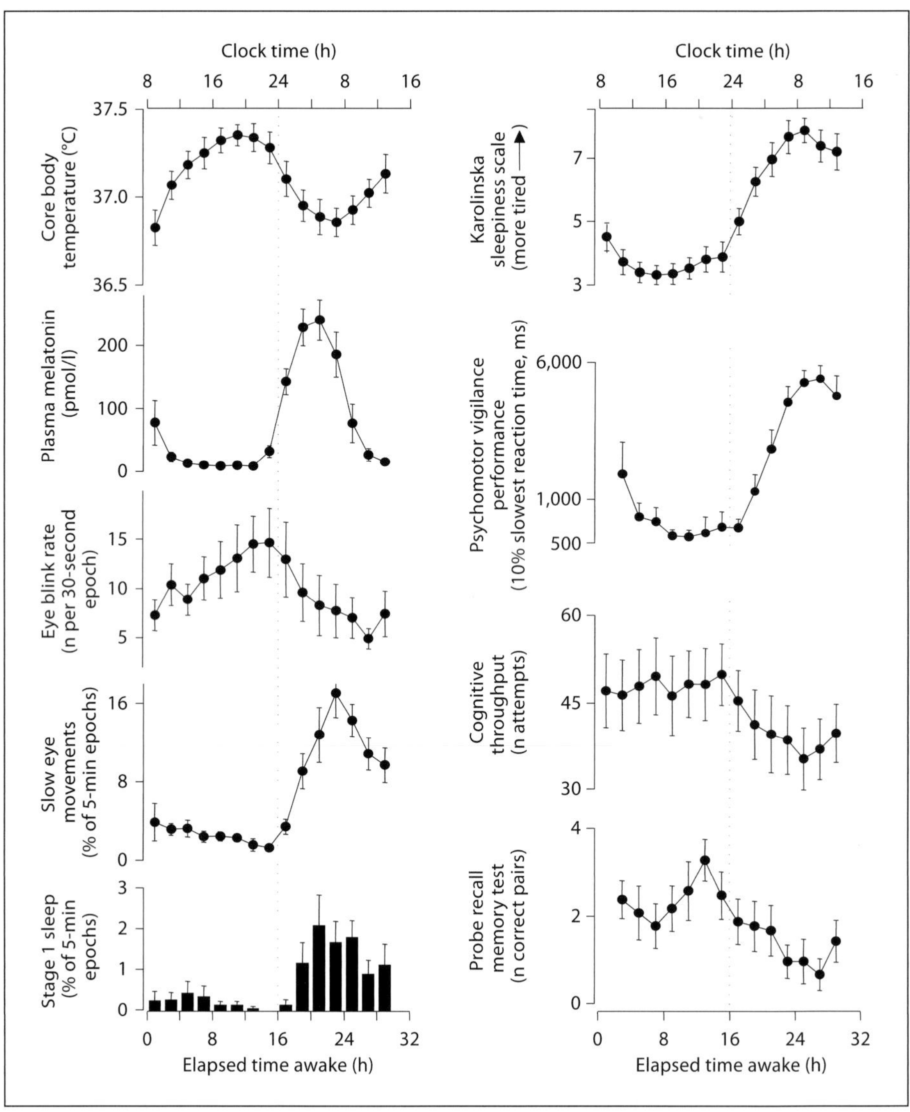

Fig. 27. Investigation of circadian and sleep-related variables measured in 10 healthy young men during 32 h of wakefulness under controlled constant routine laboratory conditions (supine posture, low light exposure, multiple isocaloric snacks). Modified from Cajochen et al. [129], with permission.

promote sleep onset (even including daytime napping in controlled experiments) [42].

Since evening melatonin administration induces a phase advance and morning melatonin a phase delay, with careful timing it can guide the circadian phase of increased sleep propensity toward the desired bedtime. Melatonin can induce sleep when the homeostatic drive to sleep (process S, section 1.4.) is insufficient, and it can also inhibit the drive for wakefulness (process C, section

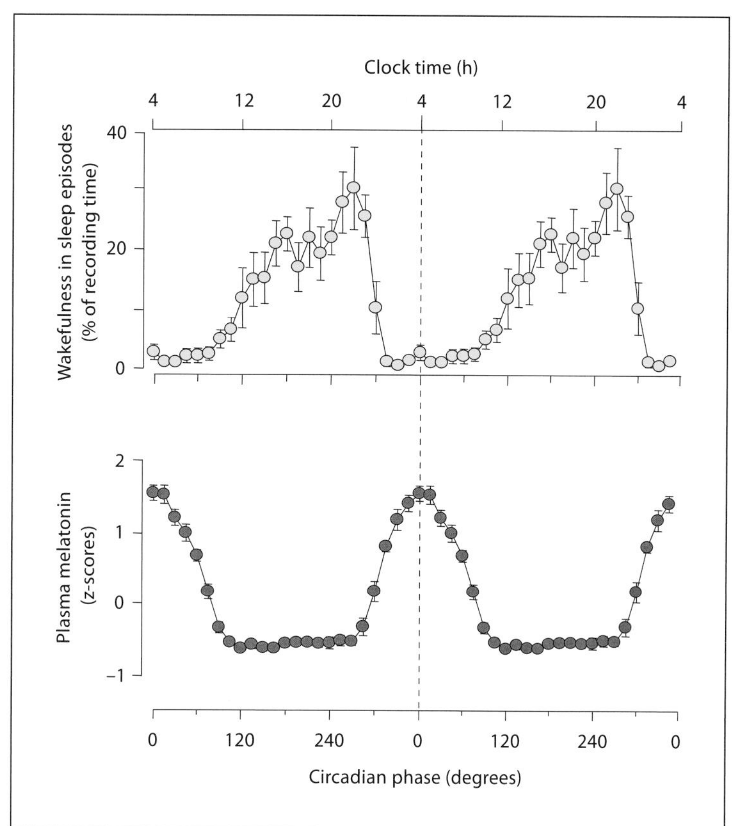

Fig. 28. The amount of wakefulness in sleep episodes depends on the circadian phase of sleep as measured by the melatonin rhythm (11 healthy young men in a forced desynchrony protocol). From Dijk et al. [130], with permission.

1.4.) that emanates from the circadian pacemaker [131]. That is why exogenous melatonin can act as soporific agent, a chronobiotic, or both.

Thermoregulatory processes have long been implicated in the initiation of human sleep. Melatonin plays a crucial role as a mediator between the thermoregulatory and arousal system [132]. Distal heat loss via increased skin temperature is intimately coupled with increased sleepiness and sleep induction. Exogenous melatonin administered during the day when melatonin is absent mimics the endogenous thermophysiological processes that occur in the evening, thereby inducing sleepiness. A topographical analysis of finger skin temperature with infrared thermometry [133] revealed that the most distal parts – e.g. the fingertips – represent the important skin regions for heat loss regulation, most probably via opening the arteriovenous anastomoses. This process is clearly potentiated by melatonin [132, 133]. Thus, warm hands and feet are the physiological gate to sleep [134]. The natural role of the evening melatonin onset of secretion is that of 'nature's soporific', to reinforce the appropriate thermoregulatory changes when the individual is ready for bed.

Interestingly, the potency of exogenous melatonin increases when the patient assumes a recumbent posture, as on the sofa or in bed. Lying down itself induces distal vasodilatation and sleepiness [132]. Such postural effects may interact with metabolism of the substance and are thus integral to dosing, a factor that should also be explored for other drugs, whether or not soporific.

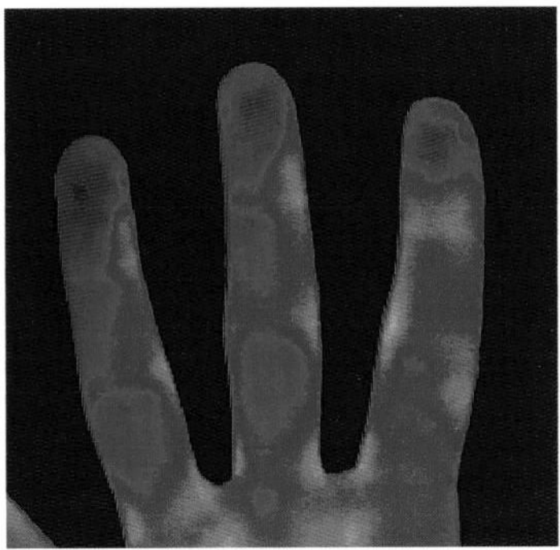

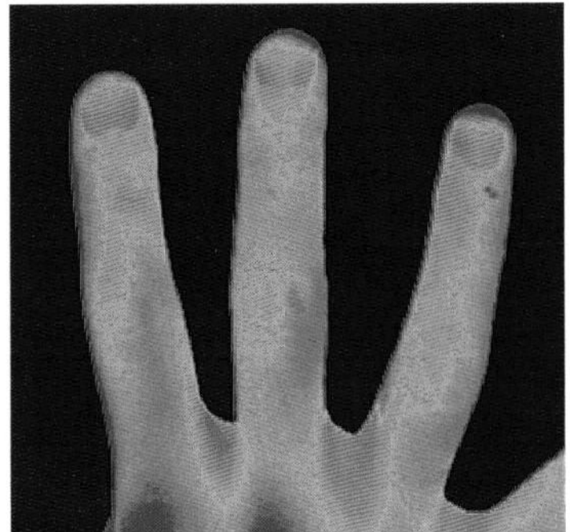

Fig. 29. Infrared thermometry of hands 1 h after administration of placebo or high-dose melatonin (5 mg) during the day, when endogenous melatonin is not produced. A similar pattern occurs naturally in the evening. Lowest temperatures are blue and green, yellow and red are warmest. The tips of the fingers show the most extreme differences in temperature. Redrawn from Kräuchi et al. [133], with permission.

12.2 Melatonin in Circadian Sleep-Wake Cycle Disturbances

These circadian and soporific effects of melatonin make it an interesting substance for treating circadian rhythm disorders and sleep onset insomnia. Treatment indications include abnormal entrainment or even failure of entrainment: delayed sleep phase disorder, a non-24-hour sleep-wake cycle (frequent in people with blindness or diminished light perception, section 11), irregular sleep-wake cycles (frequent in Alzheimer's dementia), jet lag, and shift work.

Sleep onset insomnia may, in part, be related to thermoregulatory problems – either the clock does not send out the evening signal to vasodilate at the right time, or there are circulatory problems (e.g. in older persons, or as a result of vasoconstricting medication). The circadian physiology of sleep onset as unravelled by this research shows why grandmother was right: all the old-fashioned methods to encourage a good night's sleep – a hot bath or footbath, a warm drink, hot water bottle, bedsocks – mimic the thermoregulatory changes that naturally occur.

Even lying in bed worrying, a common psychological source of sleep onset difficulties, can be explained by the simple vasoconstricting effect of enhanced alertness or stress.

Interestingly, a regimen of enhanced daytime light can increase low nocturnal melatonin to normal levels in older insomniacs, with improved sleep quality [115]. Thus, light therapy and exogenous melatonin must be considered interrelated therapeutic agents.

Melatonin – which as a natural hormone cannot be patented – is readily available as a 'food supplement' in US pharmacies and health food stores (and online), but its sale is restricted in most other countries. There is a need for tested formulations and doses that might be patented. Melatonin lies in a separate class between the weakly effective phytotherapies (such as valerian) and the powerful benzodiazepines. Melatonin appears safe in low doses, but there are no reliable data on long-term use except in blind subjects, for whom no habituation or side effects have been noted even after years of administration. Thus, potential retinal side effects have yet to be examined (the retina is a primary site of melatonergic activity) [6].

One formulation of melatonin (2.0 mg controlled release) has been tested in industry-supported clinical trials and is available in Europe for treatment of primary insomnia in older patients (www.emea.europa.eu/humandocs/Humans/EPAR/circadin/circadin.htm).

Low, physiologic doses of melatonin (0.1–0.3 mg), which introduce blood levels similar to endogenous levels, appear to be as effective or more effective than higher pharmacologic doses in promoting circadian rhythm phase advances and improved sleep latency and continuity when administered in the evening before endogenous onset [10]. Low-dose (0.3 mg) melatonin can improve polysomnographically determined sleep efficiency as effectively as a high dose (5.0 mg) administered 30 min before sleep taken during the day [131]. By contrast, common pharmacologic doses (0.5–20.0 mg) put levels into the bloodstream orders of magnitude higher than normal endogenous levels.

Because of the rapid half-life of melatonin (45–60 min), physiological doses of melatonin may wash out before their desired action is completed. One study, for example, had to administer multiple 0.1-mg doses throughout the evening in order to maintain blood levels that support circadian rhythm phase advances [135]. Controlled-release, 0.2-mg physiological-dose melatonin is under development, with a pharmacokinetic morning washout that mirrors the time course of endogenous melatonin when the tablet is taken 2 h before sleep, around the time of melatonin onset [136]. Thus, daytime overshoot of melatonin, a problem that has plagued controlled-release preparations, can be avoided. When taken in the late afternoon or early evening before endogenous melatonin onset to elicit circadian rhythm phase advances, this formulation washes out by the middle of the night, when counteracting phase delays would otherwise begin to occur (fig. 6).

It is important to recognise that the circadian and direct retinal actions of melatonin and light are antagonistic [6]. Thus, after taking melatonin, short-wavelength blue light (a major component of white light) should be avoided during daytime and evening hours in artificially illuminated environments, including the home and workplace (for shift workers). There are three considerations: (a) melatonin can have a soporific effect, while light is energizing; (b) whereas melatonin can elicit circadian rhythm phase advances when administered in late afternoon or evening before endogenous onset – and phase delays in the morning after endogenous offset – light exposure at those times has opposite effects on the circadian clock; and (c) melatonin is a suspected retinal photosensitiser [137], and thus its use outside the confines of darkness at night requires precautions (e.g. staying in dim ambient light or wearing blue-blocking glasses).

12.3 Melatonin for Depression?

Some, but not all studies of melatonin rhythms in major depression show low nocturnal secretion. Some, but not all SAD patients have a delayed melatonin phase, whereas many patients with non-seasonal depression have an earlier phase. Some, but not all antidepressants increase melatonin levels. The rationale for administering melatonin to depressed patients is therefore rather unclear. Improvements in sleep, but not in mood have been found; melatonin may be useful as adjunctive treatment for depression if rhythm abnormalities are clearly present. Two studies have investigated melatonin administration in SAD patients, however, with no antidepressant effects [87, 135] despite timing of ingestion to elicit a phase advance. In another study, melatonin reduced arousal and startle responsiveness, as might be expected from its soporific properties, but there was no direct emotion-modulating effect [138].

Although not yet formally investigated (but already successfully used clinically), evening melatonin combined with morning light appears to accelerate and strengthen circadian rhythm phase advances, thereby expediting and enhancing the antidepressant effect.

13 Drugs That Affect Rhythms (Chronobiotics)

Pharmacology and chronobiology meet in two areas. First, the effectiveness of any given medication varies with time of day it is administered (chronopharmacology) [139]. The same dose is not the same dose in the morning as at night. The time-dependent variation depends on two factors: not only do pharmacokinetics change across the daily cycle, resulting in different plasma levels of available drug, but the sensitivity of the organ or receptor system (pharmacodynamics) is also modified by time of day. Even if a drug with a longer half-life attains steady state levels, the action of the drug still varies with time of day. This is an important application of chronobiology in medicine that is only partially realised, e.g. useful for medication with a narrow efficacy/toxicity range such as anti-cancer drugs.

It is important to recognise that many antidepressants may directly or indirectly affect the circadian system [140]. If we take a simplified schematic of the circadian system (fig. 3), psychopharmacologic agents can act at several levels within or outside the system, causing changes in behavioural rhythms downstream, including the sleep-wake cycle (fig. 30). Lithium lengthens the intrinsic period of the circadian pacemaker in the SCN. It also acts on retinal photoreceptors to reduce light sensitivity. Beta-blockers diminish or entirely suppress pineal melatonin secretion – does this have indirect effects on entrainment and sleep quality? In some patients, haloperidol (dopamine antagonist) appears to diminish the amplitude of the sleep-wake cycle, whereas clozapine enhances entrainment by acting as a $5HT_7$ receptor antagonist in the SCN.

Consideration of circadian rhythm synchronisation as a drug development target is relatively new. Given that sleep disturbances often lead to depression, and that depression is accompanied by sleep disorders, an approach that focuses on normalisation of sleep and circadian rhythms is a logical step. Antidepressants may be sedating or activating, and some of them indeed cause transient insomnia.

13.1 Melatonin Agonists

Melatonin agonists with properties similar to the parent compound have therapeutic potential for the treatment of circadian rhythm sleep disorders.

Ramelteon, a selective MT1/MT2 receptor agonist, is the first in this new class of melatonergic sleep aids to be approved by the US FDA for the treatment of sleep onset insomnia. Ramelteon has both sleep-promoting and chronobiotic (zeitgeber) properties [141]. Tasimelteon (VEC-162) is a melatonin receptor agonist with high affinity for both MT1 and MT2 receptors. It has similar phase-shifting properties to melatonin, and has been shown to be effective in treating transient insomnia after a sleep-time shift [142].

Melatonin agonists offer a new medication approach to insomnia with a good safety profile. The few agonists that have undergone head-to-head comparisons with melatonin have similar chronobiotic and sleep-promoting characteristics. Although they appear to have a satisfactory safety profile, side effects may differ from the innocuous profile for melatonin (e.g. FDA safety labeling revisions for ramelteon following reports of severe anaphylactic/anaphylactoid reactions and abnormal thinking and behaviour). There are insufficient data to guide selection of

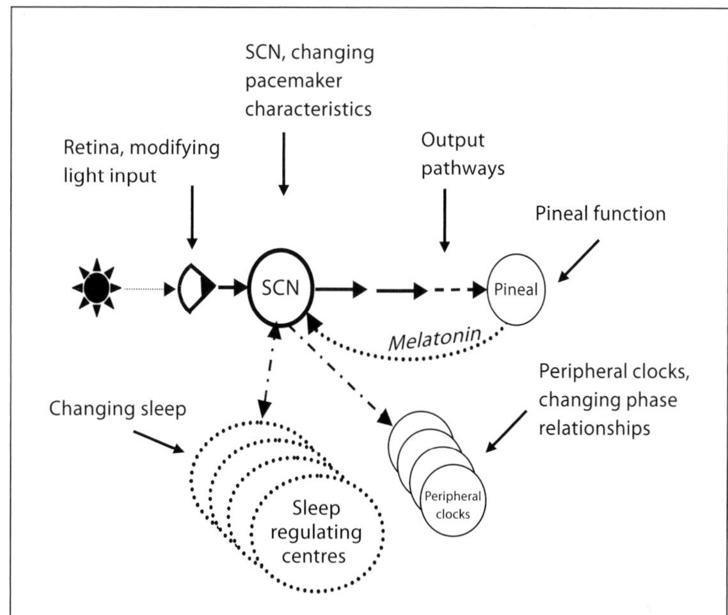

Fig. 30. Schematic of the circadian and sleep regulating systems, and where drugs could act at separate or multiple sites.

the agonists over the natural, synthesised hormone itself.

Agomelatine is a potent MT1/MT2 agonist, and also acts on the post-synaptic $5HT_{2C}$ receptor, a mechanism related to its antidepressant properties [143]. Administered in the evening, it has two characteristics similar to melatonin, acting as a zeitgeber to advance circadian phase and entrain the rhythm, and directly inducing distal vasodilation, which is the physiological gate to sleep onset [144]. In depressed patients, agomelatine promotes coalesced sleep followed by improved daytime alertness, and improves mood [145].

13.2 Chronobiology of Lithium and Antidepressants

Lithium was the first psychopharmacologic drug to be tested on circadian rhythms – *in plants*! Lithium lengthens circadian rhythm period in plant leaf movement, in hamster behaviour, and in humans studied in adventurous experiments during the Spitzbergen summer of continuous light [140]. Under entrained light-dark cycles, lithium delays circadian phase. These findings led to studies asking whether psychopharmacologic agents had a common mechanism of action in affecting the circadian pacemaker. Early animal studies suggested that antidepressants lengthened the circadian period and delayed circadian phase (e.g. the MAOI clorgyline, or the tricyclic imipramine), though follow-up investigations with a variety of antidepressants gave inconsistent results [140]. More recently, the SSRI fluoxetine produced robust phase advances of the peak of SCN neuronal activity [146], thus providing preliminary evidence that antidepressant drugs may act at the level of the circadian clock.

Studies of circadian rhythms in major depression have also yielded inconsistent results: phase variability is seen more often than any specific phase shift [2]. Thus, it is more likely that antidepressants work to stabilise phase by

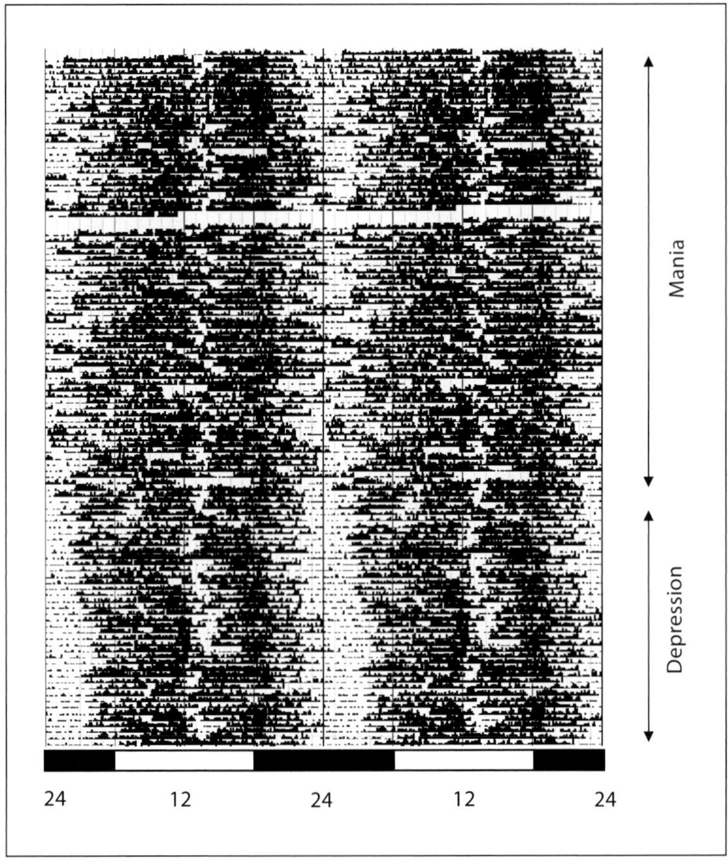

Fig. 31. Long-term actigraph recordings of the circadian rest-activity cycle in an untreated bipolar patient. The activity is shown in black, and 2 days are plotted next to one another to show the shifts in rhythm patterns more clearly (double plot). Consecutive days are also plotted beneath one another. The top half of the actigram during the manic phase shows short sleep, occasional spontaneous nights awake, early morning awakening. As clinical state shifts into depression, the rest-activity cycle shifts later, and sleep becomes longer and more consolidated. These unusual data from an unmedicated patient show that the circadian abnormalities are intrinsic to the illness and not an artefact of medication. From Cajochen, unpubl. data, with permission; see also Wehr et al. [78] for more examples.

enhancing zeitgeber strength – whether by phase advances or delays or increased amplitude of the SCN's efferent clock signals. Hence the theoretical parallel with light therapy as stabilising agent.

In bipolar disorder there is more solid evidence for a relationship of abnormal circadian phase and clinical state. The circadian rest-activity cycle is typically delayed in the depressive phase, and the switch out of depression is often associated with – perhaps even triggered by – a sleepless night [78]. During mania, sleep is short and phase advanced. Wrist actigraphy in a bipolar patient provides a striking example (fig. 31) of rhythm changes similar to those initially documented in actigraphy studies by Wehr et al. [78]. They provided convincing evidence that the spontaneous wakefulness in bipolar patients, when they switch out of depression, could be mimicked by administration of sleep deprivation. In other words, wake therapy, as we recommend for chronotherapeutics, is a very natural treatment.

13.3 Clock Genes in Depression

Although circadian rhythms have long been implicated in bipolar disorder, only recently have the genes comprising the molecular clock been discovered. Genetic evidence in bipolar patients

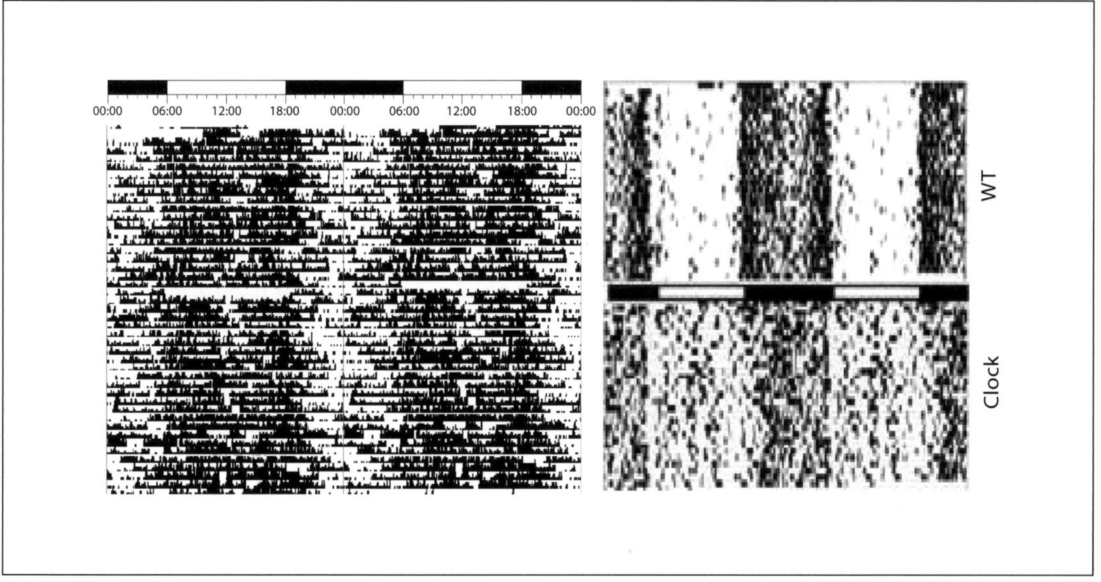

Fig. 32. Comparison of the entrained rest-activity cycle (double plotted) in untreated mania (left, from Cajochen [unpubl. data], with permission) and a Clock mutant mouse and its wild-type (WT) healthy counterpart (right, from Turek et al. [148], with permission). There is a striking similarity in the shortened, advanced rest phase with many interruptions.

suggests that the central transcriptional activator of molecular rhythms, Clock, may be particularly important [147]. Mice carrying a mutation in Clock display a behavioural profile strikingly similar to mania in humans, including hyperactivity, decreased sleep, lowered depression-like symptoms, lower anxiety, and increased reward-seeking behaviour [148]. Note the similarities between the circadian rest-activity cycle of a manic episode compared with that of a Clock mutant mouse (fig. 32).

There are also well-known links between mania and dopaminergic mechanisms. For example, a molecular link between circadian clock function and dopamine metabolism:transcription of the monoamine oxidase-A (MAOA) promoter is regulated by a number of clock components [149]. A mutation in the clock gene Per2 in mice leads to reduced expression and activity of MAOA in the mesolimbic dopaminergic system.

As of yet, no association has been found between individual variants of clock genes and depression, but common genetic polymorphisms have been shown to influence core components of the illness such as age of onset (in the case of CLOCK and hPER3) [150, 151], illness recurrence (CLOCK) [152], insomnia both for lifetime and during antidepressant treatment [150, 153], and the diurnal pattern of activity and sleep [154]. Chronotherapeutic augmentation of antidepressant medication – by wake and light therapy and sleep phase advance – enhances the rate and magnitude of response along with clock gene functional expression [77]. As research rapidly expands, we can expect to find many more molecular links to periodicity in mood disorders.

Taken together, these findings indicate that chronotherapeutics targets the biological mechanisms responsible for the unique characteristic of mood disorders – rapid switching between depression, euthymia, and mania.

A recent NIH workshop underscored the need to clarify the association between circadian oscillators and the neurotransmitter systems and brain circuits that control higher brain functions, including emotion, cognition, and social interaction (http://www.nimh.nih.gov/research-funding/scientific-meetings/2008/). Such basic research will provide new methods to chart mental illness trajectories and determine when, where and how to intervene for optimum therapeutic effect. All that said, we know enough already about environmental impacts on the circadian system for chronotherapeutics to provide major clinical benefit.

13.4 Caffeine, Modafinil

If we can treat depression by keeping patients awake for a night, what about drugs that enhance wakefulness? Amphetamine, the classic wake-promoting drug, was once used as an antidepressant. Amphetamine-like stimulants increase wakefulness by blocking dopamine reuptake and stimulating dopamine release. The dopaminergic alerting system appears involved in antidepressant action.

Caffeine, due to its stimulating effect on performance and alertness, is the classic substance to promote wakefulness. It inhibits adenosinergic receptors, which in turn are activated through GABAergic and dopaminergic interaction. Repeated small doses of caffeine during prolonged wakefulness were found to attenuate wake-dependent deterioration of cognitive performance, particularly in the second half of the night [155]. Moreover, caffeine enhanced the ability of subjects to remain consistently awake for extended periods. One clinical study of sleep deprivation has demonstrated that it keeps the patient awake without impairing the antidepressant effect [156]. Small hourly portions of coffee administered when the patient starts complaining of excessive sleepiness may be adequate to maintain wakefulness throughout the night.

Modafinil is a wake-promoting compound with low abuse potential used in the treatment of narcolepsy. Although the drug affects multiple neurotransmitter systems, dopaminergic D_1 and D_2 receptors appear essential for the arousal effect. Although modafinil does not have antidepressant properties per se, there are two potential applications in our context. First, to administer modafinil on the night of wake therapy in order to reduce the effort needed to stay awake, and to prevent microsleep and daytime naps. This combination has been used in several case studies, e.g. [157]; clinical trials are pending. Second, given that bipolar depression is commonly associated with fatigue and somnolence, adding modafinil might treat those symptoms. Several studies show adjuvant modafinil to be effective and well tolerated.

Social Rhythm Therapy

Life in our industrialised society often masks circadian rhythms that were more apparent before the advent of artificial light. We no longer live according to the natural cycle of the seasons. We can choose our day-to-day sleep and wake times according to our fancy or work demands. This contemporary lifestyle degrades the regularity and synchrony of circadian rhythms, which are so important for health and well-being. By-products of the artificial day, we say, include sleep disorders, depression and other illnesses.

Our Manual focuses on the physical zeitgeber, light, and the hormonal zeitgeber, melatonin, as exogenous agents that promote rhythmic stability and synchrony of the internal milieu with the outside world. Beyond these interventions, psychiatrists have long known and used in their daily work the therapeutic effects of carefully structuring daily activities. From the circadian rhythm point of view, strengthening daily patterns of behaviour can be clearly understood in terms of increasing zeitgeber strength. Regular daily meals are zeitgebers (in particular for peripheral clocks), as are activity and exercise. Regular social contacts at home and at work and regular work and rest schedules also contribute to rhythmic stability and amplitude.

More than 20 years ago, Ehlers et al. [158] formalised these concepts in a 'social zeitgeber' hypothesis, which described how life events disrupting an individual's normal routine could initiate a cascade that could lead to the onset of episodes of depression or mania in vulnerable individuals. They demonstrated that disruption of social rhythms is temporally associated with onset of mood episodes – particularly mania – among individuals with a history of bipolar disorder.

A psychotherapeutic intervention, interpersonal social rhythm therapy (IPSRT), specifically targets the stabilisation of daily routines in bipolar disorder. A simple daily log (Social Rhythm Metric) targets five endpoints – clock time out of bed, first contact with another person, start of work/school/volunteer/family care, dinner, bedtime – which are used as a discussion focus during therapy sessions and are quantified together in a variance measure. The protective effect of the treatment to prevent both manic and depressive episodes is related to the extent to which patients increase the regularity of their social rhythms. The same strategy promotes recovery from bipolar depression [46].

Conceptually, these psychosocial strategies extend our biological methods in that they both address the importance of good synchronisation of rhythms for mental health. They also subsume a well-known strategy in sleep medicine, sleep hygiene (with the stabilisation of bedtime and wake-up time), which may be the most critical element of IPSRT. One result of stabilising wake-up time is that morning light exposure occurs consistently – a nice by-product, which may in fact be essential to the outcome. What is missing from IPSRT in its present form – and from sleep hygiene itself – is the incorporation of structured light exposure.

15

Chronobiology in Everyday Life

15.1

Know Your Chronotype

The concept of chronotype was introduced in order to emphasise individual differences in internal clock phase relative to the day-night cycle. Chronotype reflects preferred sleep timing as well as the optimum distribution of daytime physical and mental performance. This is not a minor matter, despite light-hearted teasing of morning 'larks' and night 'owls'. In early agrarian society, 'the early bird catches the worm' had validity. Dawn and dusk delineated the work day – there was little choice but to carry out most activities in daylight. Now, in a 24/7 society that demands continuous services, we do not have to get up at dawn, yet the conventions of the past age remain, with the moral virtue of the early bird shining over the turpitude of the night owl.

It is important to recognise that we do not choose our chronotype: the largest part is genetically determined. Furthermore, chronotype changes with age [108]. The most remarkable shifts occur during adolescence, where average sleep timing drifts forward by about 15 min per year from age 12 to 20. The delay is greater for boys than girls. In girls, we have even been able to link the onset of delay shifts to menarche. After age 20, the average chronotype slowly shifts back earlier over the decades. Late chronotypes suffer varying degrees of 'social jet lag', manifested in delayed bedtimes and wake-up times as well as oversleeping on weekends in an attempt to catch up on alarm-clock-shortened sleep duration during the week [110]. Obviously, given the usual timing of school and work, the late chronotype suffers the most.

If we stratify the population for chronotype, we find significantly more depression in owls, who have the greatest difficulty in synchronising day-night rhythms with the day-night cycle. Clinicians should probe for chronotype whenever they meet a new patient. Chronotherapeutics can reduce this mismatch and the burden it creates.

15.2

Timing of School and Work Schedules versus Sleep

School times in every country have their regularity, as do normal work schedules. The range is quite small compared to the variability of chronotypes who have to fit their circadian clocks into the procrustean bed of the real world's demands.

The biologically determined delay in sleep timing with adolescence provides a serious argument for delaying the start of the school day. The additional peer pressure to stay up late may in fact reflect the delayed chronotype of this age group. The longer sleep need of younger children (9–10 h) would also be better accommodated by a later start to the school day. Current research on the role of sleep for learning and memory consolidation of the prior day's input emphasises the importance of sufficient sleep duration. By implementing delays in the school schedule, the educational establishment has an opportunity to promote daily cognitive and behavioural functioning and mental health, and perhaps even forestall the onset of mood and sleep disorders in adulthood.

Flexible work schedules (with block times for attendance) are one way to provide individuals with a time range – albeit usually small – to schedule their day to best fit their chronotype. Extreme owls usually self-select occupations that allow night work, since they are the ones that suffer most from enforced early morning job arrival. Even with a later schedule, however, owls tend toward depression and should consider bright light therapy on awakening. One psychiatrist with delayed sleep phase disorder, who could not awaken before noon and was mildly depressed, focused office hours in the evening, which appealed to many of her patients. Her goal was not to normalise her sleep schedule, and light therapy at noon served to relieve her depression. By contrast, one neuroscientist who had slept from 7 a.m. to 3 p.m. for a decade, threatened with job loss for showing up at the lab at 5 p.m., was able to normalise sleep onset to 11:30 p.m. within two weeks using an advancing schedule of low-dose, controlled release melatonin (plus blue-blockers) 4 h before sleep onset and light therapy upon awakening on a schedule of daily advances. His reaction to the change was incredulous: 'I was positive my SCN was permanently damaged!' Motivation matters.

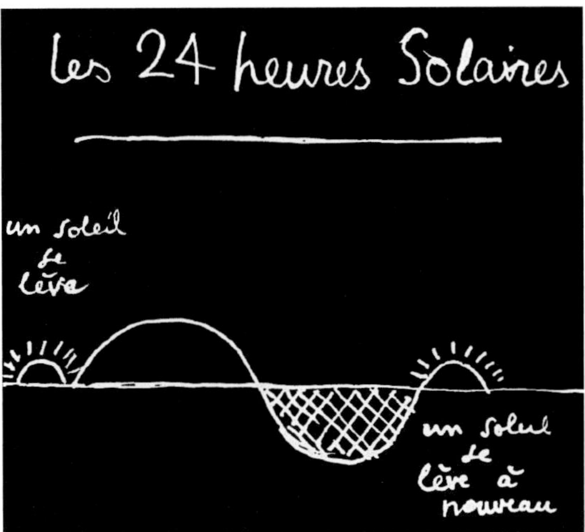

Fig. 33. The 24 solar hours, the fundamental rhythm in human life. From a lecture given in Milano, 1954. From Le Courbusier [159], p. 205, with permission. © FLC / 2009, ProLitteris, Zurich.

15.3 Light and the Built Environment: Implications for Architecture

'L'architecture est le jeu savant, correct et magnifique des volumes assemblés sous la lumière.' (Architecture is the masterly, correct and magnificent play of volumes brought together in light).

Le Corbusier: Vers une architecture, 1923

While the social clock dictates our sleep-wake schedule on work days, the built environment interacts by setting our access to daily light exposure. The intensity of room light usually lies in the range of 50–300 lx, adequate for visual perception and performance, but inadequate for maximising rhythmic stability on the desired schedule. How can we incorporate our knowledge of zeitgeber function into architectural practice? Can we implement rational light timing and intensity parameters that will work effectively depending on individual characteristics (e.g. chronotype, retinal sensitivity), or will circadian lighting installations require a compromise for the average needs of the group (workers, students, hospitalised patients)?

The principles of the circadian system and its response to light, as applied in chronotherapeutics, also directly apply to lighting design, with the aim of recapturing the biological benefits of exposure to the solar cycle. Dawn and dusk are the key signals for advancing and delaying the circadian clock, respectively; the regularity of this signal embeds sleep within the biological night and stabilises the rhythm. Light during the day is important for maintaining the amplitude of the rhythm, and a higher amplitude means better synchronisation. Thus, both appropriate timing and sufficient daytime exposure levels are necessary for healthy rhythms.

The increased incidence of sleep and depressive disorders over the last decades has of course a multitude of origins, including adverse societal pressures. From our vantage point, an obvious contributor is an urban environment that contaminates the pristine illumination pattern of the solar cycle. There is too little bright light during the day, and too much light pollution at night, reducing the day-night contrast. With deficient daylight exposure, concentration, energy, performance and mood decline.

For night-shift workers, a simplistic solution would seem to be enhanced workplace illumination, but there are explicit and unknown hazards. The major problem is that ambient bright light exposure in night shift work impinges on different chronotypes, who are differently entrained (or not, or only partially) to the work schedule. Given that the phase response curve to light (fig. 6) shifts from extreme delays to extreme advances within a short time span in the middle of the subjective night, nighttime illumination impinges unpredictably on the circadian pacemaker, leading to disturbed sleep and, essentially, mini-jet lags from day to day in either direction.

The built environment is a 24-hour presence that constrains light availability from the bedroom to the workplace and back. This is where the attention of chronobiologic-based developments should focus: dawn simulation in the bedroom, individual workplace lighting systems, dynamic lighting in schoolrooms that are differently programmed from that in old persons' homes. Although liaison between lighting manufacturers and circadian researchers has begun, it is primarily commercially driven with a rush to the sales room before the supporting data are in.

A certain flurry on the lighting scene arose with the discovery of the melanopsin photoreceptor: blue-supplemented light was patented, and bulbs with high colour temperature – e.g. 7,000 K – were inserted into lighting fixtures and recommended as superior for treating winter depression or improving school performance. Dynamic lighting systems with spectral controls were implemented by several lighting companies. After the fact, research by chronobiologists, at the behest of the industry, is attempting to justify the claims – yet many of the studies find no difference between blue-supplemented and conventional lighting systems. The interaction between classic and novel photoreceptors is complex and depends on prior light exposure conditions. Basic research is still disentangling these interactions. It is too early in the game to specify which dynamic colour sequence is suitable for which clientele, or even to specify the optimum intensity, duration and timing of protracted daytime light exposure. Despite these caveats, we do expect future research to support dynamic lighting systems with variable spectral and intensity controls for home, workplace, school, hospital and long-term care facilities – with what the shiny commercial brochures are prematurely calling 'biologically active' light.

The demands of higher intensity lighting to synchronise the biological clock may seem incompatible with energy-saving programmes. Wrong. First, the energy cost needs to be gauged against improved performance and reduced sicktime. Second, enhanced lighting regimens will need to be tailored to the needs of individual workers by use of local area controls, in distinction from ceiling installations for entire floors. Any individual will only require short exposure(s) above normal room light intensity during the work day – to jump-start the work day, to counteract the afternoon slump, and so on.

Federal and industrial lighting standards agencies are beginning to extend their purview beyond safety and minimum requirements for visual comfort and performance, to include circadian rhythm function. If this effort is to succeed, we will need an intensive R&D partnership between basic chronobiology researchers, clinicians/chronotherapists, standards agencies, architects, lighting designers and manufacturers.

References

1 Wirz-Justice A, Benedetti F, Berger M, Lam RW, Martiny K, Terman M, Wu JC: Chronotherapeutics (light and wake therapy) in affective disorders. Psychol Med 2005;35:939–944.

2 Germain A, Kupfer DJ: Circadian rhythm disturbances in depression. Hum Psychopharmacol Clin Exp 2008;23:571–585.

3 Mizukawa R, Ishiguro S, Takada H, Kishimoto A, Ogura C, Hazama H: Long-term observation of a manic-depressive patient with rapid cycles. Biol Psychiatry 1991;29:671–678.

4 Hastings MH, Maywood ES, Reddy AB: Two decades of circadian time. J Neuroendocrinol 2008;20:812–819.

5 Hankins MW, Peirson SN, Foster RG: Melanopsin: an exciting photopigment. Trends Neurosci 2008;31:27–36.

6 Remé CE, Wirz-Justice A, Terman M: The visual input stage of the mammalian circadian pacemaking system. I. Is there a clock in the mammalian eye? J Biol Rhythms 1991;6:5–29.

7 Tosini G, Pozdeyev N, Sakamoto K, Iuvone PM: The circadian clock system in the mammalian retina. Bioessays 2008;30:624–633.

8 Czeisler CA, Gooley JJ: Sleep and circadian rhythms in humans. Cold Spring Harb Symp Quant Biol 2007;72:579–597.

9 Arendt J: Melatonin and human rhythms. Chronobiol Int 2006;23:21–23.

10 Lewy AJ: Melatonin and human chronobiology. Cold Spring Harb Symp Quant Biol 2007;72:623–636.

11 Challet E: Entrainment of the suprachiasmatic clockwork in diurnal and nocturnal mammals (minireview). Endocrinology 2007;148:5648–5655.

12 Fuller PM, Gooley JJ, Saper CB: Neurobiology of the sleep-wake cycle: sleep architecture, circadian regulation, and regulatory feedback. J Biol Rhythms 2006;21:482–493.

13 Minors DS, Waterhouse JM, Wirz-Justice A: A human phase-response curve to light. Neurosci Lett 1991;133:36–40.

14 Khalsa SB, Jewett ME, Cajochen C, Czeisler CA: A phase response curve to single bright light pulses in human subjects. J Physiol 2003;549:945–952.

15 Burgess HJ, Revell VL, Eastman CI: A three pulse phase response curve to three milligrams of melatonin in humans. J Physiol 2008;586:639–647.

16 Daan S, Beersma DGM, Borbély AA: Timing of human sleep: recovery process gated by a circadian pacemaker. Am J Physiol Regulatory Integr Comp Physiol 1984;246:R161–R183.

17 Wirz-Justice A: Biological rhythm disturbances in mood disorders. Int Clin Psychopharmacol 2006;21:s11–s15.

18 Boivin DB, Czeisler CA, Dijk DJ, Duffy JF, Folkard SF, Minors DS, Totterdell P, Waterhouse JM: Complex interaction of the sleep-wake cycle and circadian phase modulates mood in healthy subjects. Arch Gen Psychiatry 1997;54:145–152.

19 Leibenluft E, Wehr TA: Is sleep deprivation useful in the treatment of depression? Am J Psychiatry 1992;149:159–168.

20 Wirz-Justice A, Van den Hoofdakker RH: Sleep deprivation in depression: what do we know, where do we go? Biol Psychiatry 1999;46:445–453.

21 Benedetti F, Barbini B, Colombo C, Smeraldi E: Chronotherapeutics in a psychiatric ward. Sleep Med Rev 2007;11:509–522.

22 Wehr TA, Rosenthal NE, Sack DA, Gillin JC: Antidepressant effects of sleep deprivation in bright and dim light. Acta Psychiatr Scand 1985;72:161–165.

23 Golden RN, Gaynes BN, Ekstrom RD, Hamer RM, Jacobsen FM, Suppes T, Wisner KL, Nemeroff CB: The efficacy of light therapy in the treatment of mood disorders: a review and meta-analysis of the evidence. Am J Psychiatry 2005;162:656–662.

24 Tuunainen A, Kripke DF, Endo T: Light therapy for non-seasonal depression (Cochrane Review); in: The Cochrane Library. Chichester, Wiley, 2004, vol 2.

25 Even C, Schröder CM, Friedman S, Rouillon F: Efficacy of light therapy in nonseasonal depression: a systematic review. J Aff Disord 2007;108:11–23.

26 Rosenthal NE, Sack DA, Gillin JC, Lewy AJ, Goodwin FK, Davenport Y, Mueller PS, Newsome DA, Wehr TA: Seasonal affective disorder: a description of the syndrome and preliminary findings with light therapy. Arch Gen Psychiatry 1984;41:72–80.

27 Terman M, Terman JS: Light therapy for seasonal and nonseasonal depression: efficacy, protocol, safety, and side effects. CNS Spectrums 2005;10:647–663.

28 Westrin A, Lam RW: Seasonal affective disorder: a clinical update. Ann Clin Psychiatry 2007;19:239–246.

29 Wirz-Justice A, Staedt J: Lichttherapie – nicht nur bei Winterdepression. Schweiz Z Psychiatr Neurol 2008;8:25–31.

30 Kripke DF, Mullaney DJ, Atkinson M, Wolf S: Circadian rhythm disorders in manic-depressives. Biol Psychiatry 1978;13:335–351.

31 Kripke DF: Light treatment for nonseasonal depression: speed, efficacy, and combined treatment. J Aff Disorders 1998;49:109–117.

32 Terman M: Evolving applications of light therapy. Sleep Med Rev 2007;11:497–507.

33 Benedetti F, Colombo C, Pontiggia A, Bernasconi A, Florita M, Smeraldi E: Morning light treatment hastens the antidepressant effect of citalopram: a placebo-controlled trial. J Clin Psychiatry 2003;64:648–653.

34 Martiny K: Adjunctive bright light in non-seasonal major depression. Acta Psychiatr Scand 2004;425(suppl):7–28.

35 Epperson CN, Terman M, Terman JS, Hanusa BH, Oren DA, Peindl KS, Wisner KL: Randomized clinical trial of bright light therapy for antepartum depression: preliminary findings. J Clin Psychiatry 2004;65:421–425.
36 Lam RW, Goldner EM, Solyom L, Remick RA: A controlled study of light therapy for bulimia nervosa. Am J Psychiatry 1994;51:744–750.
37 Blouin AG, Blouin JH, Iversen H, Carter J, Goldstein C, Goldfield G, Perez E: Light therapy in bulimia nervosa: a double-blind, placebo-controlled study. Psychiatry Res 1996;28:1–9.
38 Ancoli-Israel S, Gehrman P, Martin JL, Shochat T, Marler M, Corey-Bloom J, Levi L: Increased light exposure consolidates sleep and strengthens circadian rhythms in severe Alzheimer's disease patients. Behav Sleep Med 2003;1:22–36.
39 Fontana Gasio P, Kräuchi K, Cajochen C, Van Someren E, Amrhein I, Pache M, Savaskan E, Wirz-Justice A: Dawn-dusk simulation light therapy of disturbed circadian rest-activity cycles in demented elderly. Exp Gerontol 2003; 38:207–216.
40 Riemersma-van der Lek RF, Swaab DF, Twisk J, Hol EM, Hoogendijk WJ, Van Someren EJ: Effect of bright light and melatonin on cognitive and noncognitive function in elderly residents of group care facilities: a randomized controlled trial. JAMA 2008;299:2642–2655.
41 Goel N, Terman M, Terman JS, Macchi MM, Stewart JW: Controlled trial of bright light and negative air ions for chronic depression. Psychol Med 2005; 35:945–955.
42 Cajochen C, Kräuchi K, Wirz-Justice A: Role of melatonin in the regulation of human circadian rhythms and sleep. J Neuroedocrinol 2003;15:1–6.
43 Lockley SW, Arendt J, Skene DJ: Visual impairment and circadian rhythm disorders. Dialogues Clin Neurosci 2007;9: 301–314.
44 Wirz-Justice A, Bromundt V, Cajochen C: Circadian disruption and psychiatric disorders: the importance of entrainment. Sleep Med Clin 2009;4: in press.
45 Wehr TA, Wirz-Justice A, Goodwin FK, Duncan W, Gillin JC: Phase advance of the circadian sleep-wake cycle as an antidepressant. Science 1979;206:710–713.
46 Frank E, Soreca I, Swartz HA, Fagiolini AM, Mallinger AG, Thase ME, Grochocinski VJ, Houck PR, Kupfer DJ: The role of interpersonal and social rhythm therapy in improving occupational functioning in patients with bipolar I disorder. Am J Psychiatry 2008;165: 1559–1565.
47 Wehr TA, Turner EH, Shimada JM, Lowe CH, Barker C, Leibenluft E: Treatment of rapidly cycling bipolar patient by using extended bed rest and darkness to stabilize the timing and duration of sleep. Biol Psychiatry 1998; 43:822–828.
48 Wirz-Justice A, Quinto C, Cajochen C, Werth E, Hock C: A rapid-cycling bipolar patient treated with long nights, bedrest, and light. Biol Psych 1999;45: 1075–1077.
49 Barbini B, Benedetti F, Colombo C, Dotoli D, Bernasconi A, Cigala-Fulgosi M, Florita M, Smeraldi E: Dark therapy for mania: a pilot study. Bipolar Disord 2005;7:98–101.
50 Beauchemin KM, Hays P: Sunny hospital rooms expedite recovery from severe and refractory depressions. J Affect Disord 1996;40:49–51.
51 Benedetti F, Colombo C, Barbini B, Campori E, Smeraldi E: Morning sunlight reduces length of hospitalization in bipolar depression. J Affect Disord 2001;62:221–223.
52 Staedt J, Pless-Steinkamp C, Herfeld F, Gudlowski Y, Wirz-Justice A: Einfluss erhöhter Umgebungslichtintensität auf die Verweildauer von stationär behandelten depressiven Patienten. Nervenheilkunde 2009;28: in press.
53 Wirz-Justice A: Beginning to see the light. Arch Gen Psychiatry 1998;55: 861–862.
54 Terman JS, Terman M, Lo ES, Cooper TB: Circadian time of morning light administration and therapeutic response in winter depression. Arch Gen Psychiatry 2001;58:69–75.
55 Leibenluft E, Turner EH, Feldman-Naim S, Schwartz PJ, Wehr TA, Rosenthal NE: Light therapy in patients with rapid cycling bipolar disorder: preliminary results. Psychopharmacol Bull 1995;31:705–710.
56 Sit D, Wisner KL, Hanusa BH, Stull S, Terman M: Light therapy for bipolar disorder: a case series in women. Bipolar Disord 2007;9:918–927.
57 Weber JM, Unger I, Wirz-Justice A, Schwander JC: Supersensitive melatonin immunoassays as a tool for assessing alterations in circadian rhythms. Soc Light Treatment Biol Rhythms Abst 1998;10:178.
58 Horne JA, Ostberg O: A self-assessment questionnaire to determine morningness-eveningness in human circadian rhythms. Int J Chronobiol 1976;4:97–110.
59 Terman M, Terman JS: Controlled trial of naturalistic dawn simulation and negative air ionization for seasonal affective disorder. Am J Psychiatry 2006; 163:2126–2133.
60 Terman M, Schlager D, Fairhurst S, Perlman B: Dawn and dusk simulation as a therapeutic intervention. Biol Psychiatry 1989;25:966–970.
61 Danilenko KV, Wirz-Justice A, Kräuchi K, Weber JM, Terman M: The human circadian pacemaker can see by the dawn's early light. J Biol Rhythms 2000;15:437–446.
62 Danilenko KV, Wirz-Justice A, Kräuchi K, Cajochen C, Weber JM, Fairhurst S, Terman M: Phase advance after one or three simulated dawns in humans. Chronobiol Int 2000;17:659–668.
63 Phelps J: Dark therapy for bipolar disorder using amber lenses for blue light blockade. Med Hypotheses 2008;70: 224–229.
64 Gerner RH, Post RM, Gillin JC, Bunney WE: Biological and behavioral effects of one night's sleep deprivation in depressed patients and normals. J Psychiatr Res 1979;15:21–40.
65 Riemann D, König A, Hohagen F, Kiemen A, Voderholzer U, Backhaus J, Bunz J, Wesiack B, Hermle L, Berger M: How to preserve the antidepressive effect of sleep deprivation: a comparison of sleep phase advance and sleep phase delay. Eur Arch Psychiatry Clin Neurosci 1999;249:231–237.

66 Benedetti F, Barbini B, Campori E, Fulgosi MC, Pontiggia A, Colombo C: Sleep phase advance and lithium to sustain the antidepressant effect of total sleep deprivation in bipolar depression: new findings supporting the internal coincidence model? J Psychiatr Res 2001;35: 323–329.

67 Voderholzer U, Valerius G, Schaerer L, Riemann D, Giedke H, Schwarzler F, Berger M, Wiegand M: Is the antidepressive effect of sleep deprivation stabilized by a three day phase advance of the sleep period? A pilot study. Eur Arch Psychiatry Clin Neurosci 2003; 253:68–72.

68 Wu J, Vawter M, Bunney W, Kelsoe J, Schachat C, Demodena A: Chronotherapeutic augmentation of antidepressant medication can enhance rapidity and magnitude of response and clock genetic functional expression. Sleep Med Clin 2008;31:abstr 0409.

69 Terman M, Terman JS, Ross DC: A controlled trial of timed bright light and negative air ionization for treatment of winter depression. Arch Gen Psychiatry 1998;55:875–882.

70 Kupka RW, Altshuler LL, Nolen WA, Suppes T, Luckenbaugh DA, Leverich GS, Frye MA, Keck PE, McElroy SL, Grunze H, Post RM: Three times more days depressed than manic or hypomanic in both bipolar I and bipolar II disorder. Bipolar Disord 2007;9:531–535.

71 Altshuler L, Suppes T, Black D, Nolen WA, Keck PE, Frye MA, McElroy S, Kupka R, Grunze H, Walden J, Leverich G, Denicoff K, Luckenbaugh D, Post R: Impact of antidepressant discontinuation after acute bipolar depression remission on rates of depressive relapse at 1-year follow-up. Am J Psychiatry 2003;160:1252–1262.

72 Martiny K, Lunde M, Simonsen C, Clemmensen L, Poulsen DL, Solstad K, Bech P: Relapse prevention by citalopram in SAD patients responding to 1 week of light therapy: a placebo-controlled study. Acta Psychiatr Scand 2004;109:230–234.

73 Holsboer-Trachsler E, Hemmeter U, Hatzinger M, Seifritz E, Gerhard U, Hobi V: Sleep deprivation and bright light as potential augmenters of antidepressant drug treatment: neurobiological and psychometric assessment of course. J Psychiatr Res 1994;28:381–399.

74 Neumeister A, Goessler R, Lucht M, Kapitany T, Bamas C, Kasper S: Bright light therapy stabilizes the antidepressant effect of partial sleep deprivation. Biol Psychiatry 1996;39:16–21.

75 Benedetti F, Barbini B, Fulgosi MC, Colombo C, Dallaspezia S, Smeraldi E, Pontiggia A: Combined total sleep deprivation and light therapy in the treatment of drug-resistant bipolar depression: acute response and long-term remission rates. J Clin Psychiatry 2005; 66:1535–1540.

76 Martiny K, Refsgaard E, Lunde M, Bech P: Preliminary results from the Chronos Study: a randomized controlled trial using a combination of sleep deprivation, light therapy and sleep hygiene versus exercise in patients with major depression. Soc Light Treatment Biol Rhythms Abstr 2006;18.

77 Moscovici L, Ramat-Gan I, Kotler M: A multistage chronobiologic intervention for the treatment of depression: a pilot study. J Aff Disord 2009; in press.

78 Wehr TA, Goodwin FK, Wirz-Justice A, Breitmaier J, Craig C: 48-hour sleep-wake cycles in manic-depressive illness: naturalistic observations and sleep deprivation experiments. Arch Gen Psychiatry 1982;39:559–565.

79 Colombo C, Benedetti F, Barbini B, Campori E, Smeraldi E: Rate of switch from depression into mania after therapeutic sleep deprivation in bipolar depression. Psychiatry Res 1999;86: 267–270.

80 Benedetti F, Dallaspezia S, Fulgosi MC, Barbini B, Colombo C, Smeraldi E: Phase advance is an actimetric correlate of antidepressant response to sleep deprivation and light therapy in bipolar depression. Chronobiol Int 2007;24:921–937.

81 Terman M, Terman JS: Light therapy; in Kryger MH, Roth T, Dement WC (eds): Principles and Practice of Sleep Medicine. Philadelphia, Elsevier, 2005, 1424–1442.

82 Kuhs H, Kemper B, Lippe-Neubauer U, Meyer-Dunker J, Tölle R: Repeated sleep deprivation once versus twice a week in combination with amitriptyline. J Affect Disord 1998;7:97–103.

83 Benedetti F, Barbini B, Bernasconi A, Fulgosi MCE, Colombo C, Dallaspezia S, Lorenzi C, Pontiggia A, Radaelli D, Smeraldi E: Lithium overcomes the influence of 5-HTTLPR gene polymorphism on antidepressant response to sleep deprivation. J Clin Psychopharmacol 2008;28:249–251.

84 Pflug B: The effect of sleep deprivation on depressed patients. Acta Psychiatr Scand 1976;53:148–158.

85 Wu JC, Buchsbaum M, Bunney WE: Clinical neurochemical implications of sleep deprivation's effects on the anterior cingulate of depressed responders. Neuropsychopharmacology 2001;5: S74–S78.

86 Benedetti F, Bernasconi A, Blasi V, Cadioli M, Colombo C, Falini A, Lorenzi C, Radaelli D, Scotti G, Smeraldi E: Neural and genetic correlates of antidepressant response to sleep deprivation: a functional magnetic resonance imaging study of moral valence decision in bipolar depression. Arch Gen Psychiatry 2007;64:179–187.

87 Danilenko KV, Putilov AA: Melatonin treatment of winter depression following total sleep deprivation: waking EEG and mood correlates. Neuropsychopharmacology 2005;30:1345–1352.

88 Terman M: Blue in the face. Sleep Med 2009; Dec 22 [Epub ahead of print].

89 Terman M, Terman JS: Controlled trial of naturalistic dawn simulation and negative air ionization for seasonal affective disorder. Am J Psychiatry 2006; 163:2126–2133.

90 Lam RW: Seasonal Affective Disorder and Beyond. Light Treatment for SAD and Non-SAD Conditions. Washington, American Psychiatric Press, 1998.

91 Oren DA, Wisner KL, Spinelli M, Epperson CN, Peindl KS, Terman JS, Terman M: An open trial of morning light therapy for treatment of antepartum depression. Am J Psychiatry 2002;159: 666–669.

92 Parry BL, Curran ML, Stuenkel CA, Yokimozo M, Tam L, Powell KA, Gillin JC: Can critically timed sleep deprivation be useful in pregnancy and postpartum depressions? J Affect Disord 2000;60:201–212.

93 Parry BL, Mahan AM, Mostofi N, Klauber MR, Lew GS, Gillin JC: Light therapy of late luteal phase dysphoric disorder: an extended study. Am J Psychiatry 1993;150:1417–1419.

94 Lam RW, Carter D, Misri S, Kuan AJ, Yatham LN, Zis AP: A controlled study of light therapy in women with late luteal phase dysphoric disorder. Psychiatry Res 1999;86:185–192.

95 Parry BL, Cover H, Mostofi N, LeVeau B, Sependa PA, Resnick A, Gillin JC: Early versus late partial sleep deprivation in patients with premenstrual dysphoric disorder and normal comparison subjects. Am J Psychiatry 1995;152: 404–412.

96 Lam RW, Lee SK, Tam EM, Grewal A, Yatham LN: An open trial of light therapy for women with seasonal affective disorder and comorbid bulimia nervosa. J Clin Psychiatry 2001;62:164–168.

97 Braun DL, Sunday SR, Fornari VM, Halmi KA, et al: Bright light therapy decreases winter binge frequency in women with bulimia nervosa: a double-blind, placebo-controlled study. Compr Psychiatry 1999;40:442–448.

98 Amons PJT, Kooij JJS, Haffmans PMJ, Hoffman TO, Hoencamp E: Seasonality of mood disorders in adults with lifetime attention-deficit/hyperactivity disorder (ADHD). J Affect Disord 2006; 91:251–255.

99 Rybak YE, McNeely HE, Mackenzie BE, Jain UR, Levitan RD: Seasonality and circadian preference in adult attention-deficit/hyperactivity disorder: clinical and neuropsychological correlates. Compr Psychiatry 2007;48:562–571.

100 Rybak YE, McNeely HE, Mackenzie BE, Jain UR, Levitan RD: An open trial of light therapy in adult attention-deficit/ hyperactivity disorder. J Clin Psychiatry 2006;67:1527–1535.

101 Sloane PD, Williams CS, Mitchell CM, Preisser JS, Wood W, Barrick AL, Hickman SE, Gill KS, Connell BR, Edinger J, Zimmerman S: High-intensity environmental light in dementia: effect on sleep and activity. J Am Geriatr Soc 2007;55:1524–1533.

102 Willis GL, Turner EJ: Primary and secondary features of Parkinson's disease improve with strategic exposure to bright light: a case series study. Chronobiol Int 2007;24:521–537.

103 Demet EM, Chicz-Demet A, Fallon JH, Sokolski KN: Sleep deprivation therapy in depressive illness and Parkinson's disease. Prog Neuropsychopharmacol Biol Psychiatry 1999;23:753–784.

104 Sack RL, Auckley D, Auger RR, Carskadon MA, Wright KP, Vitiello MV, Zhdanova IV: Circadian rhythm sleep disorders. I. Basic principles, shift work and jet lag disorders: an American Academy of Sleep Medicine review. Sleep 2007;30:1460–1483.

105 Revell VL, Eastman CI: How to trick mother nature into letting you fly around or stay up all night. J Biol Rhythms 2005;20:353–365.

106 Swedo SE, Pleeter JD, Richter DM, Hoffman CL, Allen AJ, Hamburger SD, Turner EH, Yamada EM, Rosenthal NE: Rates of seasonal affective disorder in children and adolescents. Am J Psychiatry 1995;52:1016–1019.

107 Swedo SE, Allen AJ, Glod CA, Clark CH, Teicher MH, Richter D, Hoffman C, Hamburger SD, Dow S, Brown C, Rosenthal NE: A controlled trial of light therapy for the treatment of pediatric seasonal affective disorder. J Am Acad Child Adolesc Psychiatry 1997;36: 16–21.

108 Roenneberg T, Kuehnle T, Pramstaller PP, Ricken J, Havel M, Guth A, Merrow M: A marker for the end of adolescence. Curr Biol 2004;14:R1038–R1039.

109 Okawa M, Uchiyama M: Circadian rhythm sleep disorders: characteristics and entrainment pathology in delayed sleep phase and non-24-h sleep-wake syndrome. Sleep Med Rev 2007;11:485–496.

110 Wittmann M, Dinich J, Merrow M, Roenneberg T: Social jetlag: misalignment of biological and social time. Chronobiol Int 2006;23:497–509.

111 Rosenthal NE: Syndrome triad in children and adolescents. Am J Psychiatry 1995;152:1402.

112 Wasdell MB, Jan JE, Bomben MM, Freeman RD, Rietveld WJ, Tai J, Hamilton D, Weiss MD: A randomized, placebo-controlled trial of controlled release melatonin treatment of delayed sleep phase syndrome and impaired sleep maintenance in children with neurodevelopmental disabilities. J Pineal Res 2008;44:57–64.

113 Swaab DF, van Someren EJ, Zhou JN, Hofman MA: Biological rhythms in the human life cycle and their relationship to functional changes in the suprachiasmatic nucleus. Prog Brain 1996;111: 349–368.

114 Cajochen C, Münch M, Knoblauch V, Blatter K, Wirz-Justice A: Age-related changes in the circadian and homeostatic regulation of human sleep. Chronobiol Int 2006;23:461–474.

115 Mishima K, Okawa M, Shimitzu T, Hishikawa Y: Diminished melatonin secretion in the elderly caused by insufficient environmental illumination. J Clin Endocrinol Metab 2001;86:129–134.

116 Cole MG, Muller HF: Sleep deprivation in the treatment of elderly depressed patients. J Am Geriatr Soc 1976;24: 308–313.

117 Sack RL, Lewy AJ: Circadian rhythm sleep disorders: lessons from the blind. Sleep Med Rev 2001;5:189–206.

118 Sack RL, Lewy AJ, Blood ML, Keith LD, Nakagawa H: Circadian rhythm abnormalities in totally blind people: incidence and clinical significance. J Clin Endocrinol Metab 1992;75:127–134.

119 Lockley SW, Skene DJ, Arendt J, Tabandeh H, Bird AC, Defrance R: Relationship between melatonin rhythms and visual loss in the blind. J Clin Endocrinol Metab 1997;82:3763–3770.

120 Leger D, Guilleminault C, Defrance R, Domont A, Paillard M: Prevalence of sleep/wake disorders in persons with blindness. Clin Sci (Lond) 1999;97: 193–199.

121 Warman GR, Bolton C, Inglis C, Fernando A, Cheeseman J, Pawley MDM, Arendt J, Wirz-Justice A: A survey of circadian-related sleep disorders and melatonin use in the New Zealand blind population. Soc Res Biol Rhythms Abst 2008;10:88.

122 Drouyer E, Dkhissi-Benyahya O, Chiquet C, Woldemussie E, Ruiz G, Wheeler LA, Denis P, Cooper HM: Glaucoma alters the circadian timing system. PLoS ONE 2008;3:e3931. DOI: 10.1371/ journal.pone.0003931.

123 Cooper HM, Douyer E, Dkhissi-Benyahya O, Gronfier C, Chiquet C, Wolde-Mussie E, Ruiz G, Wheeler LA, Denis P: Effects of glaucoma on the circadian timing system in mice and men. Assoc Res Vision Ophthalmol Annual Meeting (ARVO-2008), Abstract 182.

124 Skalicky S, Goldberg I: Depression and quality of life in patients with glaucoma: a cross-sectional analysis using the Geriatric Depression Scale-15, assessment of function related to vision, and the Glaucoma Quality of Life-15. J Glaucoma 2008;17:546–551.
125 Banerjee A, Kumar S, Kulhara P, Gupta A: Prevalence of depression and its effect on disability in patients with age-related macular degeneration. Indian J Ophthalmol 2008;56:469–474.
126 Hahm BJ, Shin YW, Shim EJ, Jeon HJ, Seo JM, Chung H, Yu HG: Depression and the vision-related quality of life in patients with retinitis pigmentosa. Br J Ophthalmol 2008;92:650–654.
127 Ishii K, Kabata T, Oshika T: The impact of cataract surgery on cognitive impairment and depressive mental status in elderly patients. Am J Ophthalmol 2008;146:404–409.
128 Sack RL, Brandes RW, Kendall AR, Lewy AJ: Entrainment of free-running circadian rhythms by melatonin in blind people. N Engl J Med 2000;343: 1070–1077.
129 Cajochen C, Khalsa SBS, Wyatt JK, Czeisler CA, Dijk DJ: EEG and ocular correlates of circadian melatonin phase and human performance decrements during sleep loss. Am J Physiol Regulatory Integrative Comp Physiol 1999; 277:R640–R649.
130 Dijk DJ, Shanahan TL, Duffy JF, Ronda JM, Czeisler CA: Variation of electroencephalographic activity during non-rapid eye movement and rapid eye movement sleep with phase of circadian melatonin rhythm in humans. J Physiol 1997;505:851–858.
131 Wyatt JK, Dijk DJ, Ritz-de Cecco A, Ronda JM, Czeisler CA: Sleep-facilitating effect of exogenous melatonin in healthy young men and women is circadian-phase dependent. Sleep 2006; 29:609–618.
132 Kräuchi K: The thermophysiological cascade leading to sleep initiation in relation to phase of entrainment. Sleep Med Rev 2007;11:439–451.
133 Kräuchi K, Cajochen C, Pache M, Flammer J, Wirz-Justice A: Thermoregulatory effects of melatonin in relation to sleepiness. Chronobiol Int 2006;23: 475–484.
134 Kräuchi K, Cajochen C, Werth E, Wirz-Justice A: Warm feet promote the rapid onset of sleep. Nature 1999;401:36–37.
135 Lewy AJ, Lefler BJ, Emens JS, Bauer VK: The circadian basis of winter depression. Proc Natl Acad Sci USA 2006; 103:7414–7419.
136 Terman M, Hakala JC, Cooper TB, Bogner RH, Sricharoon K, Terman JS, Macchi MM, Winokur A, Oren DA: Controlled release melatonin in a physiological washout profile. Soc Light Treatment Biol Rhythms Abstr 2007; 19:29.
137 Terman M, Remé CE, Rafferty B, Gallin PF, Terman JS: Bright light therapy for winter depression: potential ocular effects and theoretical implications. Photochem Photobiol 1990;51:781–793.
138 Schachinger H, Blumenthal TD, Richter S, Savaskan E, Wirz-Justice A, Kräuchi K: Melatonin reduces arousal and startle responsiveness without influencing startle habituation or affective startle modulation in young women. Horm Behav 2008;54:258–262.
139 Lemmer B: Chronopharmakologie: Tagesrhythmen und Arzneimittelwirkung. Wissenschaftliche Verlagsgesellschaft, Stuttgart, 2004.
140 Duncan WC: Circadian rhythms and the pharmacology of affective illness. Pharmacol Ther 1996;71:253–312.
141 Sateia MJ, Kirby-Long P, Taylor JL: Efficacy and clinical safety of ramelteon: an evidence-based review. Sleep Med Rev 2008;12:319–332.
142 Rajaratnam SM, Polymeropoulos MH, Fisher DM, Roth T, Scott C, Birznieks G, Klerman EB: Melatonin agonist tasimelteon (VEC-162) for transient insomnia after sleep-time shift: two randomised controlled multicentre trials. Lancet 2008; epub. Dec. 1.
143 Millan MJ, Gobert A, Lejeune F, Dekeyne A, Newman-Tancredi A, Pasteau V, Rivet JM, Cussac D: The novel melatonin agonist agomelatine (S20098) is an antagonist at 5-hydroxytryptamine2C receptors, blockade of which enhances the activity of frontocortical dopaminergic and adrenergic pathways. J Pharmacol Exp Ther 2003;306: 954–964.
144 Kräuchi K, Cajochen C, Möri D, Graw P, Wirz-Justice A: Early evening melatonin and S-20098 advance circadian phase and nocturnal regulation of core body temperature. Am J Physiol Regulatory Integrative Comp Physiol 1997; 272:R1178–R1188.
145 Quera Salva MA, Vanier B, Laredo J, Hartley S, Chapotot F, Moulin C, Lofaso F, Guilleminault C: Major depressive disorder, sleep EEG and agomelatine: an open-label study. Int J Neuropsychopharmacol 2007;10:691–696.
146 Sprouse J, Braselton J, Reynolds L: Fluoxetine modulates the circadian biological clock via phase advances of suprachiasmatic nucleus neuronal firing. Biol Psychiatry 2006;60:896–899.
147 McClung CA: Circadian genes, rhythms and the biology of mood disorders. Pharmacol Ther 2007;114:222–232.
148 Turek F, Joshu C, Kohsaka A, Lin E, Ivanova G, McDearmon E, Laposky A, Losee-Olson S, Easton A, Jensen DR, Eckel RH, Takahashi JS, Bass J: Obesity and metabolic syndrome in circadian Clock mutant mice. Science 2005;308: 1043–1045.
149 Hampp G, Ripperger JA, Houben T, Schmutz I, Blex C, Perreau-Lenz S, Brunk I, Spanagel R, Ahnert-Hilger G, Meijer JH, Albrecht U: Regulation of monoamine oxidase A by circadian-clock components implies clock influence on mood. Curr Biol 2008;18:678–683.
150 Serretti A, Benedetti F, Mandelli L, Lorenzi C, Pirovano A, Colombo C, Smeraldi E: Genetic dissection of psychopathological symptoms: insomnia in mood disorders and CLOCK gene polymorphism. Am J Med Genet B Neuropsychiatr Genet 2003;121B:35–38.
151 Benedetti F, Dallaspezia S, Colombo C, Pirovano A, Marino E, Smeraldi E: A length polymorphism in the circadian clock gene Per3 influences age at onset of bipolar disorder. Neurosci Lett 2008; 445:184–187.
152 Benedetti F, Serretti A, Colombo C, Barbini B, Lorenzi C, Campori E, Smeraldi E: Influence of CLOCK gene polymorphism on circadian mood fluctuation and illness recurrence in bipolar depression. Am J Med Genet B Neuropsychiatr Genet 2004;123B:23–26.
153 Serretti A, Cusin C, Benedetti F, Mandelli L, Pirovano A, Zanardi R, Colombo C, Smeraldi E: Insomnia improvement during antidepressant treatment and CLOCK gene polymorphism. Am J Med Genet B Neuropsychiatr Genet 2005;137B:36–39.

154 Benedetti F, Dallaspezia S, Fulgosi MC, Lorenzi C, Serretti A, Barbini B, Colombo C, Smeraldi E: Actimetric evidence that CLOCK 3111 T/C SNP influences sleep and activity patterns in patients affected by bipolar depression. Am J Med Genet B Neuropsychiatr Genet 2007;144B:631–635.
155 Wyatt JK, Cajochen C, Ritz-de Cecco A, Czeisler CA, Dijk DJ: Low-dose repeated caffeine administration for circadian-phase-dependent performance degradation during extended wakefulness. Sleep 2004;27:374–381.
156 Schwartzhaupt AW, Lara DR, Hirakata VN, Schuch A, Almeida E, Silveira L, Caldieraro MA, Fleck MP: Does caffeine change the effect of sleep deprivation on moderate to severe depressed patients? J Affect Disord 2009;112:279–283.
157 Even C, Thuile J, Santos J, Bourgin P: Modafinil as an adjunctive treatment to sleep deprivation in depression. J Psychiatry Neurosci 2005;30:432–433.
158 Ehlers CL, Frank E, Kupfer DJ: Social zeitgebers and biological rhythms. A unified approach to understanding the etiology of depression. Arch Gen Psychiatry 1988;45:948–952.
159 Le Corbusier: The Complete Architectural Works 1957–1965, vol VII. London, Thames & Hudson, 1965.
160 Bech P, Wilson P, Wessel T, Lunde M, Fava M: A validation analysis of two self-reported HAM-D6 versions. Acta Psychiatr Scand DOI: 10.IIII/j.1600-0447.2008.01289.x.

Subject Index

N

P

R

S

T

Appendix

Appendix 1

Morningness-Eveningness self-assessment questionnaire (chronotype), with scoring and interpretation guide. © Center for Environmental Therapeutics. Automated online version: www.cet.org.

Appendix 2

Personal Inventory for Depression and SAD (diagnostic status), with scoring and interpretation. © Center for Environmental Therapeutics. Automated online version: www.cet.org.

Appendix 3

25-item expanded Hamilton Depression Scale with atypical symptoms (current level of depression), self assessment questionnaire with scoring and interpretation. © Center for Environmental Therapeutics. Automated online version and clinician administered interview version (SIGH-ADS): www.cet.org.

Appendix 4

Six-item Hamilton Depression Scale, core symptoms (for monitoring short-term changes). From [160], with permission.

Appendix 5

Daily sleep and medication logs and mood and energy ratings.

Appendix 6

Chronotherapeutics information to outpatients and clinicians following hospital discharge.

Appendix 7

Center for Environmental Therapeutics clinical assessment tools.

MORNINGNESS-EVENINGNESS QUESTIONNAIRE
Self-Assessment Version (MEQ-SA)[1]

Name: ______________________________ Date: _________________________

For each question, please select the answer that best describes you by circling the point value that best indicates how you have felt in recent weeks.

1. *Approximately* what time would you get up if you were entirely free to plan your day?

   [5] 5:00 AM–6:30 AM *(05:00–06:30 h)*
   [4] 6:30 AM–7:45 AM *(06:30–07:45 h)*
   [3] 7:45 AM–9:45 AM *(07:45–09:45 h)*
   [2] 9:45 AM–11:00 AM *(09:45–11:00 h)*
   [1] 11:00 AM–12 noon *(11:00–12:00 h)*

2. *Approximately* what time would you go to bed if you were entirely free to plan your evening?

   [5] 8:00 PM–9:00 PM *(20:00–21:00 h)*
   [4] 9:00 PM–10:15 PM *(21:00–22:15 h)*
   [3] 10:15 PM–12:30 AM *(22:15–00:30 h)*
   [2] 12:30 AM–1:45 AM *(00:30–01:45 h)*
   [1] 1:45 AM–3:00 AM *(01:45–03:00 h)*

3. If you usually have to get up at a specific time in the morning, how much do you depend on an alarm clock?

   [4] Not at all
   [3] Slightly
   [2] Somewhat
   [1] Very much

---

[1]Some stem questions and item choices have been rephrased from the original instrument (Horne and Östberg, 1976) to conform with spoken American English. Discrete item choices have been substituted for continuous graphic scales. Prepared by Terman M, Rifkin JB, Jacobs J, White TM (2001), New York State Psychiatric Institute, 1051 Riverside Drive, Unit 50, New York, NY, 10032. January 2008 version. Supported by NIH Grant MH42931. *See also:* automated version (AutoMEQ) at www.cet.org.

Horne JA and Östberg O. A self-assessment questionnaire to determine morningness-eveningness in human circadian rhythms. International Journal of Chronobiology, 1976: 4, 97-100.

MORNINGNESS-EVENINGNESS QUESTIONNAIRE
Page 2

4. How easy do you find it to get up in the morning (when you are not awakened unexpectedly)?

   [1] Very difficult
   [2] Somewhat difficult
   [3] Fairly easy
   [4] Very easy

5. How alert do you feel during the first half hour after you wake up in the morning?

   [1] Not at all alert
   [2] Slightly alert
   [3] Fairly alert
   [4] Very alert

6. How hungry do you feel during the first half hour after you wake up?

   [1] Not at all hungry
   [2] Slightly hungry
   [3] Fairly hungry
   [4] Very hungry

7. During the first half hour after you wake up in the morning, how do you feel?

   [1] Very tired
   [2] Fairly tired
   [3] Fairly refreshed
   [4] Very refreshed

8. If you had no commitments the next day, what time would you go to bed compared to your usual bedtime?

   [4] Seldom or never later
   [3] Less that 1 hour later
   [2] 1-2 hours later
   [1] More than 2 hours later

MORNINGNESS-EVENINGNESS QUESTIONNAIRE
Page 3

9. You have decided to do physical exercise. A friend suggests that you do this for one hour twice a week, and the best time for him is between 7-8 AM *(07-08 h)*. Bearing in mind nothing but your own internal "clock," how do you think you would perform?

   [4] Would be in good form
   [3] Would be in reasonable form
   [2] Would find it difficult
   [1] Would find it very difficult

10. At *approximately* what time in the evening do you feel tired, and, as a result, in need of sleep?

   [5] 8:00 PM–9:00 PM *(20:00–21:00 h)*
   [4] 9:00 PM–10:15 PM *(21:00–22:15 h)*
   [3] 10:15 PM–12:45 AM *(22:15–00:45 h)*
   [2] 12:45 AM–2:00 AM *(00:45–02:00 h)*
   [1] 2:00 AM–3:00 AM *(02:00–03:00 h)*

11. You want to be at your peak performance for a test that you know is going to be mentally exhausting and will last two hours. You are entirely free to plan your day. Considering only your "internal clock," which one of the four testing times would you choose?

   [6] 8 AM–10 AM *(08–10 h)*
   [4] 11 AM–1 PM *(11–13 h)*
   [2] 3 PM–5 PM *(15–17 h)*
   [0] 7 PM–9 PM *(19–21 h)*

12. If you got into bed at 11 PM *(23 h)*, how tired would you be?

   [0] Not at all tired
   [2] A little tired
   [3] Fairly tired
   [5] Very tired

MORNINGNESS-EVENINGNESS QUESTIONNAIRE
Page 4

13. For some reason you have gone to bed several hours later than usual, but there is no need to get up at any particular time the next morning. Which one of the following are you most likely to do?

[4] Will wake up at usual time, but will not fall back asleep
[3] Will wake up at usual time and will doze thereafter
[2] Will wake up at usual time, but will fall asleep again
[1] Will not wake up until later than usual

14. One night you have to remain awake between 4-6 AM *(04-06 h)* in order to carry out a night watch. You have no time commitments the next day. Which one of the alternatives would suit you best?

[1] Would not go to bed until the watch is over
[2] Would take a nap before and sleep after
[3] Would take a good sleep before and nap after
[4] Would sleep only before the watch

15. You have two hours of hard physical work. You are entirely free to plan your day. Considering only your internal "clock," which of the following times would you choose?

[4] 8 AM–10 AM *(08–10 h)*
[3] 11 AM–1 PM *(11–13 h)*
[2] 3 PM–5 PM *(15–17 h)*
[1] 7 PM–9 PM *(19–21 h)*

16. You have decided to do physical exercise. A friend suggests that you do this for one hour twice a week. The best time for her is between 10-11 PM *(22-23 h)*. Bearing in mind only your internal "clock," how well do you think you would perform?

[1] Would be in good form
[2] Would be in reasonable form
[3] Would find it difficult
[4] Would find it very difficult

MORNINGNESS-EVENINGNESS QUESTIONNAIRE
Page 5

17. Suppose you can choose your own work hours. Assume that you work a five-hour day (including breaks), your job is interesting, and you are paid based on your performance. At *approximately* what time would you choose to begin?

   [5] 5 hours starting between 4–8 AM *(05–08 h)*
   [4] 5 hours starting between 8–9 AM *(08–09 h)*
   [3] 5 hours starting between 9 AM–2 PM *(09–14 h)*
   [2] 5 hours starting between 2–5 PM *(14–17 h)*
   [1] 5 hours starting between 5 PM–4 AM *(17–04 h)*

18. At *approximately* what time of day do you usually feel your best?

   [5] 5–8 AM *(05–08 h)*
   [4] 8–10 AM *(08–10 h)*
   [3] 10 AM–5 PM *(10–17 h)*
   [2] 5–10 PM *(17–22 h)*
   [1] 10 PM–5 AM *(22–05 h)*

19. One hears about "morning types" and "evening types." Which one of these types do you consider yourself to be?

   [6] Definitely a morning type
   [4] Rather more a morning type than an evening type
   [2] Rather more an evening type than a morning type
   [1] Definitely an evening type

____ **Total points for all 19 questions**

MORNINGNESS-EVENINGNESS QUESTIONNAIRE
Page 6

INTERPRETING AND USING YOUR MORNINGNESS-EVENINGNESS SCORE

This questionnaire has 19 questions, each with a number of points. First, add up the points you circled and enter your total morningness-eveningness score here:

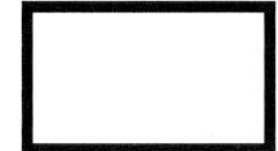

Scores can range from 16-86. Scores of 41 and below indicate "evening types." Scores of 59 and above indicate "morning types." Scores between 42-58 indicate "intermediate types."

16-30	31-41	42-58	59-69	70-86
definite evening	moderate evening	intermediate	moderate morning	definite morning

Occasionally a person has trouble with the questionnaire. For example, some of the questions are difficult to answer if you have been on a shift work schedule, if you don't work, or if your bedtime is unusually late. Your answers may be influenced by an illness or medications you may be taking. *If you are not confident about your answers, you should also not be confident about the advice that follows.*

One way to check this is to ask whether your morningness-eveningness score approximately matches the sleep onset and wake-up times listed below:

Score	16-30	31-41	42-58	59-69	70-86
Sleep onset	2:00-3:00 AM *(02:00-03:00 h)*	12:45-2:00 AM *(00:45-02:00 h)*	10:45 PM-12:45 AM *(22:45-00:45 h)*	9:30-10:45 PM *(21:30-22:45 h)*	9:00-9:30 PM *(21:00-21:30 h)*
Wake-up	10:00-11:30 AM *(10:00-11:30 h)*	8:30-10:00 AM *(08:30-10:00 h)*	6:30-8:30 AM *(06:30-08:30 h)*	5:00-6:30 AM *(05:00-06:30 h)*	4:00-5:00 AM *(04:00-05:00 h)*

If your usual sleep onset is earlier than 9:00 PM *(21:00 h)* or later than 3:00 AM *(03:00 h),* or your wake-up is earlier than 4:00 AM *(04:00 h)* or later than 11:30 AM *(11:30 h),* you should seek the advice of a light therapy clinician in order to proceed effectively with treatment.

We use the morningness-eveningness score to improve the antidepressant effect of light therapy. Although most people experience good antidepressant response to light therapy when they take a regular morning session using a 10,000 lux white light device *(see www.cet.org for recommendations)* for 30 minutes, often this will not give the best possible response. If your internal clock is shifted relative to external time (as indirectly measured by your morningness-eveningness score), the timing of light therapy needs to be adjusted.

The table at the top of the next page shows the recommended start time for light therapy for a wide range of morningness-eveningness scores. If your score falls beyond this range (either very low or very high), you should seek the advice of a light therapy clinician in order to proceed effectively with treatment.

MORNINGNESS-EVENINGNESS QUESTIONNAIRE
Page 7

Morningness-Eveningness Score	Start time for light therapy
23-26	8:15 AM
27-30	8:00 AM
31-34	7:45 AM
35-38	7:30 AM
39-41	7:15 AM
42-45	7:00 AM
46-49	6:45 AM
50-53	6:30 AM
54-57	6:15 AM
58-61	6:00 AM
62-65	5:45 AM
66-68	5:30 AM
69-72	5:15 AM
73-76	5:00 AM

If you usually sleep longer than 7 hours per night, you will need to wake up somewhat earlier than normal to achieve the effect – but you should feel better for doing that. Some people compensate by going to bed earlier, while others feel fine with shorter sleep. If you usually sleep less than 7 hours per night you will be able to maintain your current wake-up time. If you find yourself automatically waking up more than 30 minutes before your session start time, you should try moving the session later. Avoid taking sessions earlier than recommended, but if you happen to oversleep your alarm clock, it is better to take the session late than to skip it.

Our recommended light schedule for evening types – say, 8:00 AM (08:00 h) for a morningness-eveningness score of 30 – may make it difficult to get to work on time, yet taking the light earlier may not be helpful. Once you have noted improvement at the recommended hour, however, you can begin inching the light therapy session earlier by 15 minutes per day, enabling your internal clock to synchronize with your desired sleep-wake cycle and work schedule.

The personalized advice we give you here is based on a large clinical trial of patients with seasonal affective disorder (SAD) at Columbia University Medical Center in New York. Patients who took the light too late in the morning experienced only half the improvement of those who took it approximately at the times indicated. These guidelines are not only for SAD, but are also helpful in treatment of nonseasonal depression, for reducing insomnia at bedtime, and for reducing the urge to oversleep in the morning.

Our advice serves only as a *general guideline* for new users of light therapy. There are many individual factors that might call for a different schedule or dose (intensity, duration) of light. *Any person with clinical depression should proceed with light therapy only under clinical guidance.*

Reference: Terman M, Terman JS. Light therapy for seasonal and nonseasonal depression: efficacy, protocol, safety, and side effects. CNS Spectrums, 2005;10:647-663. (Downloadable at www.cet.org)

Personal Inventory for Depression and SAD
Self-Assessment Version (PIDS-SA)

This questionnaire may help you decide whether to consult a clinician about depression, whether Seasonal Affective Disorder (SAD) may be your problem, and whether treatment with light, medication or psychotherapy should be considered. This is not a method for self-diagnosis, but it can help you assess the severity and timing of certain symptoms of depression. You should answer these questions privately for your personal use and make separate copies of the questionnaire if family members or friends want to use it. Circle your responses to the right of each question, and then follow the scoring instructions.

PART 1. SOME QUESTIONS ABOUT DEPRESSION.

In the last year, have you had any single period of time lasting at least two weeks in which any of the following problems was present nearly every day? (Of course, you may also have had several such periods.)

Were there two weeks or more . . .

→ when you had trouble falling asleep or staying asleep, or sleeping too much?	***YES***	***NO***
→ when you were feeling tired or had little energy?	***YES***	***NO***
→ when you experienced poor appetite or overeating? Or significant weight gain or loss, although you were not dieting?	***YES***	***NO***
→ when you found little interest or little pleasure in doing things?	***YES***	***NO***
→ when you were feeling down, depressed, or hopeless?	***YES***	***NO***
→ when you were feeling bad about yourself — or that you were a failure — or that you were letting yourself or your family down?	***YES***	***NO***
→ when you had trouble concentrating on things, like reading the newspaper or watching television?	***YES***	***NO***
→ when you were so fidgety or restless that you were moving around a lot more than usual? Or the opposite — moving or speaking so slowly that other people could have noticed?	***YES***	***NO***
→ when you were thinking a lot about death or that you would be better off dead, or even thinking of hurting yourself?	***YES***	***NO***

How many questions above did you score "yes"? ____

PART 2. HOW 'SEASONAL' A PERSON ARE YOU?

Circle one number on each line to indicate how much each of the following behaviors or feelings changes with the seasons. (For instance, you may find you sleep different hours in the winter than in the summer.)

(0 = no change, 1 = slight change, 2 = moderate change, 3 = marked change, 4 = extreme change.)

Change in your total sleep length (including nighttime sleep and naps)	*0*	*1*	*2*	*3*	*4*
Change in your level of social activity (including friends, family and co-workers)	*0*	*1*	*2*	*3*	*4*
Change in your general mood, or overall feeling of well-being	*0*	*1*	*2*	*3*	*4*
Change in your weight	*0*	*1*	*2*	*3*	*4*
Change in your appetite (both food cravings and the amount you eat)	*0*	*1*	*2*	*3*	*4*
Change in your energy level	*0*	*1*	*2*	*3*	*4*

What's the sum total of the numbers you circled above? ____

-2-

PART 3. WHICH MONTHS STAND OUT AS 'EXTREME' FOR YOU?

For each of the following behaviors or feelings, draw a circle around all applicable months. If no particular month stands out for any item, circle "none". You should circle a month only if you recollect a distinct change in comparison to other months, occurring for several years. You may circle several months for each item.

COLUMN A

I tend to feel worst in

Jan Feb Mar Apr May Jun July Aug Sep Oct Nov Dec none

I tend to eat most in

Jan Feb Mar Apr May Jun July Aug Sep Oct Nov Dec none

I tend to gain most weight in

Jan Feb Mar Apr May Jun July Aug Sep Oct Nov Dec none

I tend to sleep most in

Jan Feb Mar Apr May Jun July Aug Sep Oct Nov Dec none

I tend to have the least energy in

Jan Feb Mar Apr May Jun July Aug Sep Oct Nov Dec none

I tend to have the lowest level of social activity in

Jan Feb Mar Apr May Jun July Aug Sep Oct Nov Dec none

COLUMN B

I tend to feel best in

Jan Feb Mar Apr May Jun July Aug Sep Oct Nov Dec none

I tend to eat least in

Jan Feb Mar Apr May Jun July Aug Sep Oct Nov Dec none

I tend to lose most weight in

Jan Feb Mar Apr May Jun July Aug Sep Oct Nov Dec none

I tend to sleep least in

Jan Feb Mar Apr May Jun July Aug Sep Oct Nov Dec none

I tend to have the most energy in

Jan Feb Mar Apr May Jun July Aug Sep Oct Nov Dec none

I tend to have the highest level of social activity in

Jan Feb Mar Apr May Jun July Aug Sep Oct Nov Dec none

For Column A and Column B above, how many times did you circle each month?

	Jan	*Feb*	*Mar*	*Apr*	*May*	*Jun*	*Jul*	*Aug*	*Sep*	*Oct*	*Nov*	*Dec*	*NONE*
COLUMN A	___	___	___	___	___	___	___	___	___	___	___	___	___
COLUMN B	___	___	___	___	___	___	___	___	___	___	___	___	___

PART 4. MORE ABOUT POSSIBLE WINTER SYMPTOMS . . .

In comparison to other times of the year, during the winter months, which — if any — of the following symptoms tend to be present?

I tend to sleep longer hours (napping included).	***YES***	***NO***
I tend to have trouble waking up in the morning.	***YES***	***NO***
I tend to have low daytime energy, feeling tired most of the time.	***YES***	***NO***
I tend to feel worse, overall, in the late evening than in the morning.	***YES***	***NO***
I tend to have a distinct temporary slump in mood or energy in the afternoon.	***YES***	***NO***
I tend to crave more sweets and starches.	***YES***	***NO***
I tend to eat more sweets and starches, whether or not I crave them.	***YES***	***NO***
I tend to crave sweets, but mostly in the afternoon and evening.	***YES***	***NO***
I tend to gain more weight than in the summer.	***YES***	***NO***

How many questions above did you score "yes"? ____

Personal Inventory for Depression and SAD
Self-Assessment Version (PIDS-SA)

Michael Terman, PhD, and Janet B.W. Williams, DSW
New York State Psychiatric Institute and
Department of Psychiatry, Columbia University

INTERPRETATION GUIDE

Part 1. If you circled five or more problems, it is possible that you have had a major depressive disorder for which you should consider seeking help. Even if you circled only one or two problems you may want to consult with a psychiatrist, psychologist, social worker or other mental health professional if the problems worry you or interfere with your daily activities. You may have experienced some of these problems for *less* than two weeks — if so, your problem is probably not a "major" depressive disorder (as clinically defined), but still may be serious enough to merit consultation with a therapist, and possible treatment. To determine whether the problem might be seasonal, consider Parts 2 and 3 below.

Part 2. If your total score on Part 2 is less than 6, you fall within the "nonseasonal" range. You probably do not have seasonal affective disorder (SAD). If your score on Part 1 was high, however, it is still possible that you have experienced a depression that merits the attention and guidance of a mental health professional.

If your score on Part 2 falls between 7 and 11, you may have a mild version of SAD for which seasonal changes are noticeable, and possibly even quite bothersome. If your score is 12 or more, SAD that is clinically significant is increasingly likely. But you still need to consider which months pose most problems, as shown in Part 3.

Part 3. People with *fall or winter* depression tend to score 4 or more per month in a series of 3-5 months beginning anytime between September and January, as would be noted in Column A. For months outside that range the score tends to be zero, or nearly zero. In Column B, the same people will usually score 4 or more points per month over a series of 3-5 months beginning anytime between March and June.

Some people show a different pattern, with scores divided between Columns A and B during both winter and summer months. For example, they may feel worst and socialize least during the summer, especially July and August; during that same period, they may eat least, lose most weight, and sleep least. In winter, they may feel best and socialize most, yet still tend to eat most, gain most weight, and sleep most. Such people may experience seasonal depression of the *summer* type, and treatment recommendations will differ from those for winter depression.

Some people show *relatively* high scores in the fall and winter months in Column A (winter depression), but there is also a scatter of good and bad months *throughout* the year. Such a pattern may indicate a winter worsening of symptoms, rather than clear-cut SAD. Recommendations for winter treatment might be similar to those for winter SAD, although there may be a need for additional treatments.

Some people experience depression in the winter as well as in the summer, but they feel fine in the spring and the fall. In contrast with the winter, their summer depression is usually not accompanied by oversleeping and overeating. This is a special case of SAD, for which different treatments might be appropriate in winter and summer. Even people who experience only winter depression sometimes feel summertime slumps in mood and energy when the weather is rainy or dark for several days. They often find relief by brief use of their winter treatment during these periods.

Part 4. If you reported any of these specific behaviors, you have experienced winter symptoms that may respond to treatments for SAD, regardless of whether or not you have depressed mood. The higher your score in Part 4, the more likely you are to have winter SAD. It is possible, however, to be depressed in winter *without* these symptoms — or even with *opposite* symptoms such as reduced sleep and appetite. If so, a mental health professional might recommend a treatment not designed specifically for SAD

NOTES

For further information about SAD and its treatments, see the website of the Center for Environmental Therapeutics, www.cet.org.

Part 1 was adapted from the *Prime-MD Clinician Evaluation Guide*, developed by Robert L. Spitzer, MD, and Janet B.W. Williams, DSW, New York State Psychiatric Institute and Department of Psychiatry, Columbia University. Parts 2 and 3 were adapted from the *Seasonal Pattern Assessment Questionnaire* developed by Norman E. Rosenthal, MD, Gary J. Bradt, and Thomas A. Wehr, MD, National Institute of Mental Health. Preparation of the PIDS was sponsored in part by Grant MH42930 from the U.S. National Institute of Mental Health to the Research Foundation for Mental Hygiene, New York State Psychiatric Institute.

SELF-REPORT SUMMARY (SIGH-SAD-SA 2008)

Date ___ ___ / ___ ___ / ___ ___

In the questions that follow, please circle the number of one alternative in each set that best describes how you have been during the past week, and enter the rating in the left-hand columns (Group A or Group B). If you have changed during the last few days, circle the alternative that best describes how you are today. Before you select an alternative in each set, read all of the choices to make sure you pick the most accurate one.

GROUP A RATINGS	GROUP B RATINGS	
Rating: ☐		**DURING THE PAST WEEK . . .** QUESTION 1 0 - I have ***not*** been feeling down or depressed at all. 1 - I have been feeling somewhat down or depressed. 2 - I have been feeling quite down or depressed. 3 - I have been feeling and looking very depressed (or others have said so). 4 - I haven't been able to think about anything except how bad or depressed I feel.
Rating: ☐		QUESTION 2 0 - I have been keeping busy and have been interested in the things I've been doing. 1 - I haven't been quite as interested in doing things as I used to be. 2 - I have definitely not been as interested in things as I used to be, and I have had to push myself to do them. 3 - I have not been doing much because I feel so bad. 4 - I have stopped doing nearly everything — I just sit or sleep most of the day.
	Rating: ☐	***Note: When an item refers to how you "normally" are, it means when you are feeling OK, or as close to OK as you get.*** QUESTION 3 0 - I have been interested in socializing with others as much as normal. 1 - I have still been interacting with others but am less interested in doing so. 2 - I have been interacting less with other people in social situations. 3 - I have been interacting less with others at home or at work. 4 - I have become quite withdrawn at home or at work.
Rating: ☐		QUESTION 4 ***(This question is about your interest in sex, not your actual sexual activity.)*** 0 - My interest in sex has been about the same as it was before I became depressed, or greater than normal. 1 - I have not been quite as interested in sex as I was before I became depressed. 2 - I have been much less interested in sex than I was before I became depressed.

The SIGH-SAD Self-Assessment version (SIGH-SAD-SA) is based on a self-rated depression inventory *(SIGH-SAD-SR)* developed by J.B.W. Williams, D.S.W., M.J. Link, B.S., and M. Terman, Ph.D. In turn, the SIGH-SAD-SR was based on the *Structured Interview Guide for the Hamilton Depression Rating Scale - Seasonal Affective Disorder Version (SIGH-SAD),* by J.B.W. Williams, M.J. Link, N.E. Rosenthal, and M. Terman (1998), New York, New York State Psychiatric Institute. The work was supported in part by BRSG Grant 903-E759S from the Research Foundation for Mental Hygiene, Inc., and the U.S. National Institute of Mental Health Grant MH-42931.

Rating: ☐		***Remember, "normal" means how you're feeling when you're OK.*** QUESTION 5 0 - My appetite has been normal or greater than normal. 1 - I have had less appetite than normal, but I eat without anyone having to urge me. 2 - I have had so little appetite that I have not been eating regularly unless someone urges me to.
Rating: ☐		QUESTION 6 ***(Circle "0" for this question if you have lost weight due to dieting, or have lost weight that you had previously gained when you were depressed.)*** 0 - I don't think I have lost any weight since I became depressed, or if I have lost weight, I have started to gain it back. 1 - I have probably lost some weight (that I haven't gained back at all) because I haven't felt like eating. 2 - I have definitely lost weight (that I haven't gained back at all) because I haven't felt like eating.
	Rating: ☐	QUESTION 7 0 - I have ***not*** gained weight above my normal level in the past week. 1 - I have probably gained weight (two or more pounds) in the past week, and my current weight is above normal for me. 2 - I have definitely gained weight (two or more pounds) in the past week, and my current weight is above normal for me.
	Rating: ☐	QUESTION 8 ***(This question is about your appetite, not what you have actually been eating.)*** 0 - My appetite has been normal or less than normal. 1 - I have wanted to eat just a little more than normal. 2 - I have wanted to eat somewhat more than normal. 3 - I have wanted to eat much more than normal.
	Rating: ☐	QUESTION 9 ***(This question is about what you have actually been eating.)*** 0 - I have ***not*** been eating more than normal. 1 - I have been eating a little more than normal. 2 - I have been eating somewhat more than normal. 3 - I have been eating much more than normal.
	Rating: ☐	QUESTION 10 0 - I have ***not*** been craving or eating sweets or starches any more than when I feel normal. 1 - I have been craving or eating sweets or starches somewhat more than when I feel normal. 2 - I have been craving or eating sweets or starches much more than when I feel normal. 3 - I have had an irresistible craving for sweets or starches.
Rating: ☐		QUESTION 11 0 - I have ***not*** had any difficulty falling asleep at night. 1 - Some nights it has taken me longer than half an hour to fall asleep. 2 - I have had trouble falling asleep every night.

SIGH-SAD-SA, Page 2

<table>
<tr><td>Rating:
☐</td><td></td><td>QUESTION 12
0 - I have not been waking up in the middle of the night, or if I have gotten up to go to the bathroom, I have fallen right back asleep.
1 - My sleep has been restless and disturbed during the night.
2 - I have been waking during the night without being able to get right back to sleep, or I've been getting out of bed in the middle of the night (not just to go to the bathroom).</td></tr>
<tr><td>Rating:
☐</td><td></td><td>QUESTION 13
0 - I have been oversleeping or waking up at a reasonable hour in the morning.
1 - I have been waking up very early in the morning, but I have been able to go back to sleep.
2 - I have been waking up very early in the morning without being able to go back to sleep, especially if I've gotten out of bed.</td></tr>
<tr><td></td><td>Rating:
☐</td><td>Remember, "normal" means how you're feeling when you're OK.

QUESTION 14
When I am feeling normal, I usually sleep about ___ hours each day, including naps.

0 - I have been sleeping no more than I usually do when I feel normal.
1 - I have been sleeping at least one hour more than I usually do when I feel normal.
2 - I have been sleeping at least two hours more than I usually do when I feel normal.
3 - I have been sleeping at least three hours more than I usually do when I feel normal.
4 - I have been sleeping at least four hours more than I usually do when I feel normal.</td></tr>
<tr><td></td><td></td><td>QUESTION 15
0 - I have not had a heavy feeling in my limbs, back or head.
1 - I have had a heavy feeling in my limbs, back, or head, some of the time.
2 - I have had a heavy feeling in my limbs, back, or head, a lot of the time.</td></tr>
<tr><td></td><td></td><td>QUESTION 16
0 - I have not been bothered by backaches, headache, or muscle aches.
1 - I have been bothered some of the time by backaches, headache, or muscle aches.
2 - I have been bothered a lot of the time by backaches, headache, or muscle aches.</td></tr>
<tr><td>Overall rating for Questions 15-17:
☐
See instructions below:</td><td>Rating for Question 17:
☐</td><td>Remember, "normal" means how you're feeling when you're OK.

QUESTION 17
0 - I have not been feeling more tired than normal.
1 - I have felt slightly more tired than normal.
2 - I have been more tired than normal for at least a few hours per day.
3 - I have felt tired much of the time most days.
4 - I have felt an overwhelming fatigue all of the time.</td></tr>
<tr><td colspan="3">To find your "overall rating," first identify which of Questions 15, 16 and 17 had the highest rating. If your highest rating was a "2", enter your overall rating as a "1". If the highest rating was a "3" or "4" on Question 17, enter your overall rating as a "2". Otherwise, just enter your highest uncorrected score, "0", "1" or "2".</td></tr>
</table>

SIGH-SAD-SA, Page 3

Rating:		QUESTION 18 0 - I have ***not*** been putting myself down, or feeling like a failure or that I have let other people down, or feeling guilty about things I have done. 1 - I have been feeling like a failure or that I have let other people down. 2 - I have been feeling very guilty or thinking a lot about bad things I have done, or bad mistakes I have made. 3 - I believe that my being depressed is a punishment for something bad that I've done. 4 - I have been hearing voices accusing me of bad things, or seeing things that are scary, that others said were not really there.
Rating:		QUESTION 19 0 - I have ***not*** had any thoughts about dying or about hurting or killing myself, or that life is not worth living. 1 - I have had thoughts that life is not worth living, or that I'd be better off dead. 2 - I have thought about dying, or wish I were dead. 3 - I have thought about killing myself, or I have done something to hurt myself. 4 - I have tried to kill myself.
Rating:		QUESTION 20 0 - I have ***not*** been feeling especially tense or irritable, or worrying a lot. 1 - I have been feeling somewhat tense or irritable. 2 - I have been worrying about little unimportant things — that I wouldn't ordinarily worry about — or I have been excessively tense or irritable. 3 - Other people notice that I look or sound tense, anxious, or fearful. 4 - I feel tense, anxious, or fearful all of the time.
		Check off all the following physical symptoms that have <u>bothered</u> you in the past week: *_dry mouth* *_cramps* *_hyperventilating* *_gas* *_belching* *_sighing* *_indigestion* *_heart palpitations* *_having to urinate frequently* *_diarrhea* *_headaches* *_sweating*
Rating:		QUESTION 21 ***Referring to the physical symptoms listed above:*** 0- I didn't check off any symptoms above. 1 - Altogether, the symptom(s) have only been bothering me a little bit. 2 - Altogether, the symptom(s) have been bothering me somewhat. 3 - Altogether, the symptom(s) have been bothering me a lot. 4 - Altogether, the symptom(s) have been making it difficult for me to function.
Rating:		QUESTION 22 0 - I have ***not*** been thinking much about my physical health. 1 - I have been worrying about being or becoming physically ill. 2 - I have been spending most of my time worrying about my physical health. 3 - I have been complaining frequently about how I feel physically, or asking for help a lot. 4 - I am sure that I have a physical disease, even though the doctors tell me that I don't. ***Have you had a specific medical problem this week? If yes, please describe:*** ____ ***Have you taken any medications in the past week? If yes, please describe:*** ____

SIGH-SAD-SA, Page 4

Rating: ☐		*Remember, "normal" means how you're feeling when you're OK.* QUESTION 23 0 - My rate of speech and thought are normal. 1 - My speech and physical movements are slightly slowed down, or my thoughts are slightly slower, which has made it difficult for me to concentrate. 2 - My physical movements, speech or thoughts are somewhat slow compared to normal, and other people have noticed this. 3 - My physical movements are markedly slower, or my speech or thoughts are so slow that it has been hard to have a conversation with me. 4 - My physical movements are greatly slowed down, or my speech and thoughts are so slow that it has been difficult for me to think or talk at all.
Rating: ☐		QUESTION 24 0 - I have ***not*** been restless or fidgety. 1 - I have been somewhat restless, or sometimes have been playing with my hands, hair, or other things. 2 - I have been very restless, or often have been playing with my hands, hair, or other things. 3 - I have trouble sitting still, and need to keep moving about a lot of the time. 4 - I am unable to sit still, or have been wringing my hands, biting my nails, pulling my hair, or biting my lips, nearly all the time.
		In the following question, a "slump" means a <u>temporary</u> reduction in mood or energy from which you recover, at least partially, later in the day. 0 - I have ***not*** regularly had a slump in my mood or energy in the afternoon or evening. 1 - I have regularly had a slump in my mood or energy in the afternoon or evening. ***If you circled "1" for the question above, please also specify:*** 0 - Once these slumps occur, they usually last until bedtime. 1 - I usually come out of these slumps at least an hour before bedtime.
	Rating: ☐	QUESTION 25 ***Please circle the best description of slumps you may be experiencing:*** 0 - I do not have such slumps, or my slumps last until bedtime. 1 - Usually, the temporary slumps have been only mild in intensity. 2 - Usually, the temporary slumps have been moderate in intensity. 3 - Usually, the temporary slumps have been severe in intensity.

TOTAL OF GROUP A RATINGS:	**TOTAL OF GROUP B RATINGS:**	**GRAND TOTAL OF ALL RATINGS (A+B):**	***In the spaces to the left, add up your ratings for Group A (column 1) and Group B (column 2), and the grand total of all your ratings (Groups A and B).***
☐	☐	☐	

INTERPRETING AND ACTING ON YOUR QUESTIONNAIRE RESULTS

SIGH-SAD-SA

In the sections below, please use the left-hand boxes to write your corresponding ratings from the questionnaire, and then consider how your answers fit with the interpretation and recommendations. If your rating does not fall in to the range specified, skip that section and continue below. For example, on the first three sections, if your grand total score is higher than 4, leave the boxes blank and skip down to find the boxes that apply to you.

Grand total = 0 to 4 ↓	Question 1 Rating ↓	▪ **Q1 = 0:** depression is probably not a current concern. ▪ **Q1 = 2 to 3:** you reported feeling down, but without many of the usual symptoms of depression. Use the questionnaire again next week – hopefully this is temporary. ▪ **Q1 = 4:** you reported that you are feeling very depressed even without many of the symptoms that indicate clinical depression. You should talk with someone close about it. If the feeling lasts, you should seek a clinician's guidance.
Grand total = 0 to 4 ↓	Question 2 Rating = 2 to 4 ↓	▪ **Q2 = 2 or 3:** you reported loss of interest or engagement in activities, without having many of the symptoms that indicate clinical depression. Use the questionnaire again next week – hopefully this is temporary. ▪ **Q2 = 4:** you reported that you have lost interest in or are not engaging in usual activities without many of the symptoms that indicate clinical depression. Hopefully this is temporary, but you should talk with someone close about it. If the feeling lasts, you should seek a clinician's guidance.
Grand total = 0 to 4 ↓	Question 19 rating = 1 to 4 ↓	▪ **Q19 = 1 or 2:** you reported thoughts of death or suicide. This is rare but possible if you do not feel otherwise depressed. Check www.befrienders.org for help worldwide. These services are all free and confidential. Remember, our questionnaire was designed to help you identify problems, but you have to take the next step to solve them. ▪ **Q19 = 3 or 4:** you reported intentions of suicide. This is possible, although it does not ordinarily accompany otherwise mild depression. If you are actively thinking about suicide, try to tell someone close about it and go to the nearest emergency room for help or dial your emergency number (for example, 911). Check www.befrienders.org for help worldwide. These services are all free and confidential. Remember, our questionnaire was designed to help you identify problems, but you have to take the next step to solve them.
Grand total = 5 to 10 ↓	Question 1 Rating ↓	▪ Your rating indicates that you are experiencing depressive symptoms at a mild level. Hopefully this is temporary, but you should talk with someone close about it. If the feeling lasts, you should seek a clinician's guidance. ▪ **Q1 = 0:** you also reported, however, that your mood has been normal for you, while low mood is a central symptoms of depression. It is possible that your symptoms reflect another problem, for example, physical illness or a sleep disorder.
Grand total = 5 to 10 ↓	Question 19 Rating = 1 to 4 ↓	▪ **Q19 = 1 or 2:** Apart from your report of mild depression, you also reported thoughts of death or suicide. This is possible, although it does not ordinarily accompany otherwise mild depression. Check www.befrienders.org for help worldwide. Remember, our questionnaire was designed to help you identify problems, but you have to take the next step to solve them. ▪ **Q19 = 3 or 4:** Apart from your report of mild depression, you also reported intentions of suicide. This is possible, although it does not ordinarily accompany otherwise mild depression. If you are actively thinking about suicide, try to tell someone close about it and go to the nearest emergency room for help or dial your emergency number (for example, 911). Check www.befrienders.org for help worldwide. These services are all free and confidential. Remember, our questionnaire was designed to help you identify problems, but you have to take the next step to solve them.

SIGH-SAD-SA, Page 6

Grand total = 11 to 19 ↓	Question 19 Rating ↓	▪ Your ratings indicates that you are experiencing depressive symptoms at a moderate level. If you have not already done so, you should talk with someone close about it. This may require clinical attention if it lasts as long as two weeks. ▪ **Q19 = 1 or 2:** you also reported thoughts of death or suicide. It is very important that you get guidance from a clinician. Try to tell someone close about it and check www.befrienders.org for help worldwide. These services are all free and confidential. Remember, our questionnaire was designed to help you identify problems, but you have to take the next step to solve them. ▪ **Q19 = 3 or 4:** you also reported intentions of suicide. It is very important that you get prompt guidance from a clinician. If you are actively contemplating suicide, try to tell someone close about it and go to the nearest emergency room for help or dial your local emergency number (for example, 911). Check www.befrienders.org for help worldwide. Remember, our questionnaire was designed to help you identify problems, but you have to take the next step to solve them.
Grand total = 20 or above ↓	Question 19 Rating ↓	▪ Your ratings indicates that you are experiencing clinically significant depressive symptoms. If you have not already done so, you should talk with someone close about it and seek the guidance of clinician if this has lasted longer than a week. ▪ **Q19 = 1 or 2:** you also reported thoughts of death or suicide. It is very important that you get guidance from a clinician. Try to tell someone close about it and check www.befrienders.org for help worldwide. These services are all free and confidential. Remember, our questionnaire was designed to help you identify problems, but you have to take the next step to solve them. ▪ **Q19 = 3 or 4:** you also reported intentions of suicide. It is very important that you get prompt guidance from a clinician. If you are actively contemplating suicide, try to tell someone close about it and go to the nearest emergency room for help or dial your local emergency number (for example, 911). Check www.befrienders.org for help worldwide. Remember, our questionnaire was designed to help you identify problems, but you have to take the next step to solve them.
Grand total = 10 to 15 ↓	Group B rating = 10 or above ↓	▪ You reported a set of symptoms – which might include fatigue, oversleeping and food cravings – that can be quite severe even without depressed mood. Morning light therapy might be helpful.
Question 11 Rating = 2 ↓		▪ You reported having trouble falling asleep every night. Although this kind of insomnia can accompany depression, it can be troublesome even when someone is not depressed. Sleep disorders can arise for many reasons. Hopefully this is temporary, but if the problem lasts, you should report this to your doctor.
Question 12 Rating = 2 ↓		▪ You reported waking during the night (not just to go to the bathroom). Although this kind of insomnia can accompany depression, it can be troublesome even when someone is not depressed. Sleep disorders can arise for many reasons. Hopefully this is temporary, but if the feeling lasts, you should report this to your doctor.
Question 13 Rating = 2 ↓		▪ You reported waking up too early without being able to go back to sleep. Although this kind of insomnia can accompany depression, it can be troublesome even when someone is not depressed. Sleep disorders can arise for many reasons. Hopefully this is temporary, but if the problem lasts, you should report this to your doctor.
Question 18 Rating = 4 ↓		▪ You reported being bothered by voices accusing you of bad things, or having scary visions. Even if this is temporary or infrequent, you should seek a clinician's guidance.
Question 20 Rating = 3 or 4 ↓		▪ You reported feeling tense, anxious or fearful. Although this feeling often accompanies depression, it can be troublesome even when someone is not depressed. Hopefully this is temporary, but if the feeling lasts, you should seek a clinician's guidance.

SIGH-SAD-SA, Page 7

Question 21 Rating = 4 ↓		▪ You reported one or more physical symptoms that have been making it difficult for you to function. You should report this to your doctor if this does not pass quickly.
Question 23 Rating = 3 or 4 ↓		▪ You reported that your physical movements, speech or thought have been greatly slowed down. Although this often happens during depression, it can be troublesome even when someone is not depressed. You should report this to your doctor.
Question 24 Rating = 4 ↓		▪ You reported being unable to sit still or acting very nervously. Although this often happens during depression, it can be troublesome even when someone is not depressed. You should report this to your doctor.

Development team: Michael Terman Ph.D., Janet B.W. Williams D.S.W., Thomas M. White M.D., Madeleine Gould Ph.D., Department of Psychiatry, Columbia University and New York State Psychiatric Institute, New York, NY 10032 USA. *January 2008 version.*

SIGH-SAD-SA, Page 8

The HAM-D_6 Questionnaire

In this questionnaire you will find six groups of statements. Please choose the one statement in each group that best describes how you have been feeling over the past three days, including today, and mark it with an **X** in the corresponding box.

(1) *During the past three days*

I have been in my usual good mood		0
I have felt a little more sad than usual		1
I have been clearly more sad than usual, but haven't felt helpless or hopeless		2
I have been so gloomy that I briefly have felt overpowered by hopelessness		3
I have been so low in my moods that everything seems dark and hopeless		4

(2) *During the past three days*

I have been quite satisfied with myself		0
I have been a little more self-critical than usual with a tendency to feel less worthy than others		1
I have been brooding over my failures in the past		2
I have been plagued with distressing guilt feelings		3
I have been convinced that my current condition is a punishment		4

(3) *During the past three days*

My daily activities have been as usual		0
I have been less interested in my usual activities		1
I have felt that I have had difficulty performing my daily activities, but I was still able to perform them with great effort		2
I have had difficulty performing even simple routine activities		3
I have not been able to do any of the most simple day-to-day activities without help		4

(4) *During the past three days*

I have felt neither restless nor slowed down		0
I have felt a little slowed down		1
I have felt rather slowed down or have been talking a little less than usual		2
I have felt clearly slowed down or subdued or have talked much less than usual		3
I have hardly been talking at all or felt extremely slowed down all the time		4

(5) *During the past three days*

I have been calm and relaxed		0
I have felt a little more tense or insecure than usual		1
I have been clearly more worried or tense than usual, but have not felt that I lost control		2
I have been so tense or worried that I have briefly I felt close to panic		3
I have had episodes where I was overwhelmed by panic		4

(6) *During the past three days*

I have been as active and have had as much energy as usual		0
I have felt rather low in energy or physically unwell with some bodily pains		1
I have felt very low in energy or had bodily pains		2

DAILY SLEEP/MOOD/ENERGY LOG

INTRUCTIONS

1. Enter your name and the start date for this sheet.
2. After you wake up for the day, fill in 15-minute sleep intervals. If awake at night for 15 minutes or more, leave box blank. *Use your best recollection:* you should not be checking the clock while you are trying to sleep. Also mark daytime naps.
3. Enter the letter "L" (for light) at the time to your light therapy session, if you are using lights.
4. Enter a symbol at appropriate times for medications and melatonin ("M" for melatonin). Define symbols on the list to the right.
5. For multiple medications taken at the same time, enter a "1", "2" or "3" at appropriate times, as shown on the list to the right.
6. In the morning, when you record your sleep, enter average mood and energy ratings for *yesterday*.
7. Enter notes to explain unusual situations (for example, "out late," "stomach ache").
8. *Women:* if you are menstruating, add a note for each day.

IDENTIFY MEDICATIONS/DOSES TAKEN ONE OR MORE TIMES OF DAY, OR "PRN" (AS NEEDED). SPECIFY A SYMBOL FOR EACH DRUG.

1 - Morning: ____________________

2 - Midday: ____________________

3 - Evening: ____________________

4 - PRN: ____________________

NAME: ____________________ **START DATE:** _____ / _____ / _____

DAILY RATINGS
0 - worst ever
5 - feeling OK, fine
10 - highest ever

SUNDAY PM 12 1 2 3 4 5 6 7 8 9 10 11 (noon) — **MONDAY AM** 12 1 2 3 4 5 6 7 8 9 10 11 (midnight)

NOTES (place at time): ____________________

Sunday's *mood* ☐ *energy* ☐

MONDAY PM 12 1 2 3 4 5 6 7 8 9 10 11 (noon) — **TUESDAY AM** 12 1 2 3 4 5 6 7 8 9 10 11 (midnight)

NOTES: ____________________

Monday's *mood* ☐ *energy* ☐

TUESDAY PM 12 1 2 3 4 5 6 7 8 9 10 11 (noon) — **WEDNESDAY AM** 12 1 2 3 4 5 6 7 8 9 10 11 (midnight)

NOTES: ____________________

Tuesday's *mood* ☐ *energy* ☐

WEDNESDAY PM 12 1 2 3 4 5 6 7 8 9 10 11 (noon) — **THURSDAY AM** 12 1 2 3 4 5 6 7 8 9 10 11 (midnight)

NOTES: ____________________

Wednesday's *mood* ☐ *energy* ☐

THURSDAY PM 12 1 2 3 4 5 6 7 8 9 10 11 (noon) — **FRIDAY AM** 12 1 2 3 4 5 6 7 8 9 10 11 (midnight)

NOTES: ____________________

Thursday's *mood* ☐ *energy* ☐

FRIDAY PM 12 1 2 3 4 5 6 7 8 9 10 11 (noon) — **SATURDAY AM** 12 1 2 3 4 5 6 7 8 9 10 11 (midnight)

NOTES: ____________________

Friday's *mood* ☐ *energy* ☐

SATURDAY PM 12 1 2 3 4 5 6 7 8 9 10 11 (noon) — **SUNDAY AM** 12 1 2 3 4 5 6 7 8 9 10 11 (midnight)

NOTES: ____________________

Saturday's *mood* ☐ *energy* ☐

Start a new page for next week.

CONTINUING LIGHT THERAPY AT HOME AFTER CHRONOTHERAPEUTICS IN HOSPITAL

A Guide for Outpatients and their Clinicians

In hospital, the patient underwent a course of chronotherapeutics to regularize circadian rhythms and sleep as an adjunct to antidepressant or mood stabilizing treatment. Components of chronotherapeutics include wake therapy (one or more nights abstaining from sleep), light therapy and sleep phase advance therapy (earlier sleep time on the days following wake therapy. The regimen is adjusted for each individual, and not everyone undergoes all three procedures. The common element is light therapy, usually scheduled at a preset wake-up time somewhat earlier than during the depressive episode.

The background and procedures are explained in: Wirz-Justice A, Benedetti F, and Terman M (2009) *Chonotherapeutics for Affective Disorders: A Clinician's Manual for Light and Wake Therapy*, Basel, Karger. The manual is available at www.cet.org, the nonprofit website of the Center for Environmental Therapeutics.

Light therapy is a maintenance treatment that should continue at home after hospital discharge. If the light box is not provided by the hospital when the patient leaves, one should be purchased for prompt use upon the transition home. For information on light box selection, also see www.cet.org.

Light therapy presents a full dose of daylight-level illumination, most often for 15 to 60 minutes shortly after awakening. The patient sits at the light box, which projects light downward toward the head, and engages in any compatible sedentary activity, such as reading, writing, laptop, iPod, and having breakfast. Eyes must remain open. Although the patient does not look directly at the screen, it is important to face forward for an even distribution of illumination.

Depending on the expected episode course (seasonal, nonseasonal recurrent, or chronic) daily maintenance is recommended until the end of April (for winter depression) or for up to one year. After several weeks of home treatment, if the depression remains remitted, the patient can test the effect of skipping a day of light therapy now and then. Some patients will notice an immediate slump, while others can coast for several days or longer before resuming treatment. If the patient shows mood worsening when treatment is skipped, the original effect can almost always be recaptured after resumption for several days. If the clinician expects the episode has entirely passed, it may be possible to discontinue light therapy for a longer term (*e.g.,* May to September in cases of winter depression, or until an unanticipated episode recurrence).

The dosing of light therapy is comprised of three dimensions: light intensity (high/low setting on the light box, or seating distance from the light box), duration of the session, and time of day of the treatment session. These three factors interact, and may have to be adjusted during the course of maintenance treatment. For example, a seasonal patient who has responded well in December to 30 minute sessions at 10,000 lux, at 7 AM, may require 45 minutes in January and February, when symptoms peak. Too high a dose can result in autonomic hyperactivation (*e.g.,* agitation) or switching in patients with bipolar disorder. The experienced light therapy patient develops a keen sense for adequate light dose, but should consult or notify the clinician when a dose change seems indicated.

It is useful for both patient and clinician to keep a systematic weekly or biweekly record of mood state throughout the course of light therapy (and after) to track trends of improvement or symptom recurrence. An online questionnaire at www.cet.org, the *AutoSIGH* (based on the expanded Hamilton Rating Scale) returns a score summary with individualized interpretation, which can be printed out by the patient for monitoring by the clinician.

Clinical Assessment Tool Collection

Center for Environmental Therapeutics

CET's clinical assessment tools were designed and produced by the Clinical Chronobiology and Biometrics Research groups at Columbia University's Psychiatric Institute. The instruments provide state-of-the-art structured interviews for clinicians to rate the severity of depression (including atypical symptoms) and hypomania, and self-rating versions for patients to complete for clinician review. In addition, there is a diagnostic interview for Atypical Depression keyed to DSM-IV-TR criteria for atypical features, and a paper-and-pencil version of the Morningness-Eveningness Questionnaire also presented in an on-line automated version on this website. For patients considering light therapy, there is a structured eye-screening chart for completion by optometrists and ophthalmologists, and a sleep log to help in specifying the prescribed interval for light therapy. For use after treatment begins, we offer a comprehensive questionnaire for monitoring side effects.

Readers of *Chronotherapeutics for Affective Disorders* may access the collection free of charge from the Clinicians section at www.cet.org by entering the following password: ***colleagues***.

PACKET CONTENTS

Personal Inventory for Depression and SAD (PIDS), with scoring and interpretation guide. Surveys the presence of symptoms of depression, using a validated diagnostic algorithm (PRIME-MD). Also probes for seasonal pattern of the symptoms and presence of atypical neurovegetative features. An interpretation guide is included for use by clinicians in patient pre-screening. Can be completed in the waiting room or sent to prospective patients.

Personal Inventory for Depression and SAD - Self-Assessment Version (PIDS-SA), with scoring and interpretation guide, to help determine whether a clinical consultation for SAD is indicated.

Structured Interview Guide for the Hamilton Depression Rating Scale with Atypical Depression Supplement (SIGH-ADS). Designed for general use in depression research and clinical evaluation, regardless of seasonality. The questions have greater specificity those in the predecessor **SIGH-SAD** (also included) and the flow of questioning is distinctly smoother. The SIGH-ADS rates the severity of depressive symptoms in terms of Hamilton's 17- and 21-item depression scales and the NIMH/Columbia addendum of eight atypical symptoms.

Self-Report Summary [Structured Interview Guide for the Hamilton Depression Rating Scale - Seasonal Affective Disorder Version. Self-Rating Version (SIGH-SAD-SR)], with scoring and interpretation guide for clinicians. This version can be used as a stand-alone instrument for outpatient monitoring, or for reliability checks against interviewer ratings on the SIGH-SAD.

Depression Self-Assessment inventory (SIGH-SAD-SA). Scoring algorithm generates detailed scale and symptom assessment for self-monitoring of current state or preparation for office visits.

Hypomania Interview Guide (including Hyperthymia) - Current Assessment Version (HIGH-C). The HIGH-C measures the pattern and severity of symptoms that characterize hyperthymia, hypomania, and mania. A subset of the items can be used to provide a provisional DSM-IV diagnosis of current Hypomanic Episode or lifetime Bipolar II disorder.

Self-Report Summary [Hypomania Interview Guide (including Hyperthymia) - Current Assessment Version. Self-Rating Version (HIGH-C-SR)], with combined instruction guide for the HIGH instruments. Especially useful for outpatient monitoring.

Hypomania Interview Guide (including Hyperthymia) - Retrospective Assessment Version (HIGH-R), with DSM-IV scoring algorithm and interpretation guide. The HIGH-R provides a provisional lifetime diagnosis irrespective of current clinical state.

Diagnostic Interview for Atypical Depression (DIAD), including instruction and interpretation guide. The DIAD is a structured interview that allows the rater to assess atypical symptoms of depression based on both DSM-IV and Columbia criteria. This instrument was designed to ease questioning on the sensitive issue of rejection sensitivity and to increase the specificity and reliability of the diagnosis.

Morningness-Eveningness Questionnaire (MEQ) of Horne and Östberg (revised for smooth presentation in "American English"). As illustrated by the feedback section of the automated version (AutoMEQ) on this website, the instrument is used to gauge circadian rhythm phase (in a reflection of melatonin onset) and derive the optimum timing for morning light therapy.

Morningness-Eveningness Questionnaire - Self-Assessment Version (MEQ-SA), with score interpretation guide and circadian phase estimate for timing of light therapy.

The Columbia Eye Check-Up for Users of Light Treatment, a structured chart for ophthalmologists and optometrists to determine whether there are any contraindications for use of bright light therapy or periodic monitoring is indicated.

Systematic Assessment for Treatment Emergent Effects (SAFTEE) - Self-Rating Version. A checklist adaptation of the comprehensive NIMH interview, used to detect and monitor side effects of light, negative air ion or drug treatment.

Daily Sleep Log and Mood/Energy Ratings for monitoring pre- and posttreatment patterns, and determining and adjusting the timing of light treatment for optimum response. At Columbia's Center for Light Treatment and Biological Rhythms, all inpatients and outpatients maintain this log for weekly review of progress, side effects (such as fractionated sleep and early-morning awakening), compliance/adherence and scheduling.

Authors

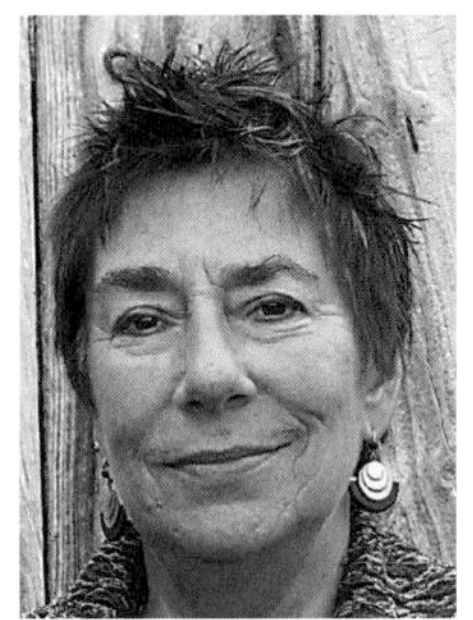

Anna Wirz-Justice PhD (University College London 1967) is emeritus Professor of Psychiatric Neurobiology at the Centre for Chronobiology, Psychiatric University Clinics Basel. Her research focuses on human circadian and seasonal rhythms and sleep regulation, sleep deprivation and light therapy for depression.

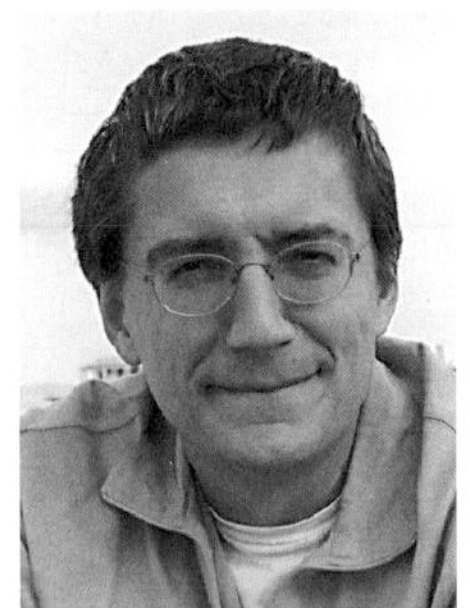

Francesco Benedetti MD (University of Modena 1991) is Head of the Psychiatry and Clinical Neurosciences research unit at the San Raffaele Hospital in Milano, and contract professor at the University Vita-Salute San Raffaele. His research ranges from clinical chronotherapeutics of mood disorders, to neuroimaging and genetics of psychiatric diseases and therapeutics.

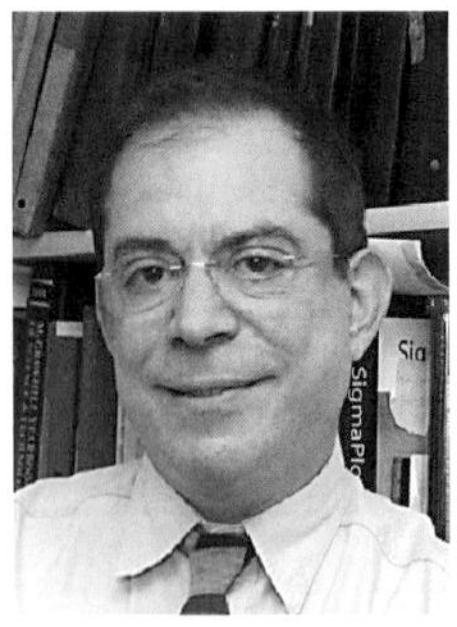

Michael Terman PhD (Brown University 1968) is Professor of Clinical Psychology in Psychiatry at Columbia University's College of Physicians & Surgeons. His research has encompassed photobiology and circadian rhythms in animal models; clinical chronobiology (light, melatonin and negative air ionisation therapy for depressive and sleep disorders); and instrumentation development for chronotherapeutics.